The Sociology of Healthcare Safety and Quality

Sociology of Health and Illness Monograph Series

Edited by Professor Ian Rees Jones
Cardiff School of Social Sciences
WISERD
46 Park Place
Cardiff
CF10 3BB
Wales, UK

The Sociology of Healthcare Safety and Quality

Edited by

Davina Allen, Jeffrey Braithwaite, Jane Sandall
and Justin Waring

WILEY Blackwell

This edition first published 2016
Originally published as Volume 38, Issue 2 of *The Sociology of Health & Illness*
Chapters © 2016 The Authors.
Book Compilation © 2016 Foundation for the Sociology of Health & Illness/Blackwell Publishing Ltd.

Blackwell Publishing was acquired by John Wiley & Sons in February 2007. Blackwell's publishing program has been merged with Wiley's global Scientific, Technical, and Medical business to form Wiley Blackwell.

Registered Office
John Wiley & Sons Ltd, The Atrium, Southern Gate, Chichester, West Sussex, PO19 8SQ, United Kingdom

Editorial Offices
350 Main Street, Malden, MA 02148-5020, USA
9600 Garsington Road, Oxford, OX4 2DQ, UK
The Atrium, Southern Gate, Chichester, West Sussex, PO19 8SQ, UK

For details of our global editorial offices, for customer services, and for information about how to apply for permission to reuse the copyright material in this book please see our website at www.wiley.com/wiley-blackwell.

The rights of Davina Allen, Jeffrey Braithwaite, Jane Sandall and Justin Waring to be identified as the authors of the editorial material in this work has been asserted in accordance with the UK Copyright, Designs and Patents Act 1988.

Wiley also publishes its books in a variety of electronic formats. Some content that appears in print may not be available in electronic books.

Designations used by companies to distinguish their products are often claimed as trademarks. All brand names and product names used in this book are trade names, service marks, trademarks or registered trademarks of their respective owners. The publisher is not associated with any product or vendor mentioned in this book. This publication is designed to provide accurate and authoritative information in regard to the subject matter covered. It is sold on the understanding that the publisher is not engaged in rendering professional services. If professional advice or other expert assistance is required, the services of a competent professional should be sought.

Library of Congress Cataloging-in-Publication Data is available for this book.

ISBN 9781119276340

A catalogue record for this book is available from the British Library.

Set in 9.5/11.5pt TimesNewRomanMTStd by Aptara Inc., New Delhi, India
Printed and bound in Malaysia by Vivar Printing Sdn Bhd

1   2016

Contents

Notes on contributors

Davina Allen School of Healthcare Sciences, Cardiff University, UK

Emma-Louise Aveling Department of Health Sciences, University of Leicester, UK; Department of Health Policy and Management, Harvard T.H. Chan School of Public Health, Boston, USA

Jeffrey Braithwaite Australian Institute of Health Innovation, Macquarie University, Australia

Patrick R. Brown Department of Sociology and Centre for Social Science and Global Health, University of Amsterdam, The Netherlands

Michael W. Calnan School of Social Policy, Sociology and Social Research, University of Kent

Stephen Campbell NIHR Greater Manchester Patient Safety Translational Research Centre (GM PSTRC), NIHR School for Primary Care Research, University of Manchester & Research and Action in Public Health (CeRAPH), University of Canberra

Gavin Daker-White NIHR Greater Manchester Patient Safety Translational Research Centre (GM PSTRC), University of Manchester

Huw Davies School of Management, University of St. Andrews, UK

Mary Dixon-Woods Department of Health Sciences, University of Leicester, UK

Tim Freeman Leadership, Work and Organisation, Middlesex University, UK

Suzanne Grant Division of Population Health Sciences, University of Dundee, Scotland

Bruce Guthrie Division of Population Health Sciences, University of Dundee, Scotland

Nicola Mackintosh Division of Women's Health, King's College London, London, UK

Russell Mannion Health Services Management Centre, Birmingham, UK

Ruth McDonald Manchester Business School and NIHR School for Primary Care Research, University of Manchester

Jessica Mesman Faculty of Arts and Social Sciences, Department of Technology and Society Studies, Maastricht, the Netherlands

Ross Millar   Health Services Management Centre, Birmingham, UK

Michael Parker   Ethox Centre, University of Oxford, UK

Penny Rhodes   NIHR School for Primary Care Research, University of Manchester

Jane Sandall   Division of Women's Health, King's College London, London, UK; Women's Health Academic Centre, King's College London, UK

Caroline Sanders   NIHR School for Primary Care Research & Manchester Academic Health Sciences Centre (MAHSC), University of Manchester

Julia E. Szymczak   Division of Infectious Diseases and The Center for Pediatric Clinical Effectiveness, The Children's Hospital of Philadelphia, USA

Justin Waring   Nottingham University Business School, University of Nottingham, UK

1

Towards a sociology of healthcare safety and quality
Davina Allen, Jeffrey Braithwaite, Jane Sandall and Justin Waring

Introduction

Improving the quality and safety of healthcare is a global priority (Braithwaite *et al.* 2015, WHO 2002). As healthcare organisations and systems across the developed and developing world face unprecedented financial constraints, growing demands for services (especially from ageing populations with long-term conditions and co-morbidities), and the challenge of keeping pace with technological progress, the case for a deeper understanding of these issues is particularly pressing. Hitherto, research and practice in quality and safety have been dominated by disciplines such as medical and safety science, social psychology, and human factors which have framed how quality and safety is understood, how it should be measured and studied, and the policies, interventions and practices through which it should be addressed. While quality and safety cuts across many traditional sociological concerns, and sociology has continued to progress understanding in this field, its insights and potential contribution have, until recently, been relatively neglected by mainstream policy and research. This might, in part, reflect a tension between the interventionist orientation of proponents of the dominant paradigm and the more critical detached stance of sociologists who, historically at least, have eschewed simplistic explanations or prescriptions for policy and practice. It may also arise from the complexities so often revealed by sociological research, rendering pressing clinical and organisational problems as less amenable to immediate solutions. After all sociologists have the reputation of Cassandra: when we make prophesies they are usually laden with doom and thus fated to be disregarded (Dingwall and Allen 2001). It is also the case that while sociologists have made, and continue to make, important contributions to the understanding of quality and safety, much of this work is fragmented across different sub-specialisms. As the introductory review chapter to this monograph shows (Waring *et al.* this volume), the insights of classic contributions by Strauss *et al.* (1985) on the social organisation of healthcare work, Illich (1976) on medical iatrogenesis, Bosk (1979) on managing medical mistakes, Timmermans and Berg (1997) on standardization, Fox (1999) on medical uncertainty and Rosenthal (1995) on the management of problematic doctors have largely been ignored within the prevailing orthodoxy. Within sociology itself, however, these earlier studies have provided the foundations for a new generation of sociological research oriented to this policy priority (for example, Dixon-Woods 2010, Jensen 2008, Mol 2008, Waring 2005). What has emerged from this growing corpus of work is a recognition that patient safety is not simply a matter of individual or group psychology or systems engineering,

The Sociology of Healthcare Safety and Quality, First Edition. Edited by Davina Allen, Jeffrey Braithwaite, Jane Sandall and Justin Waring. Chapters © 2016 The Authors. Book Compilation © 2016 Foundation for the Sociology of Health & Illness/Blackwell Publishing Ltd.

but is shaped by wider socio-cultural and political structures. A sociological perspective also reveals the hidden influence of inequalities of power (between occupations, within occupations and between patients and professionals) on quality and safety, how these problems might be managed and by whom, as well as the everyday – and often invisible – situated practices through which quality and safety are accomplished (Allen 2014, Iedema *et al.* 2006, Mackintosh and Sandall 2010, Macrae 2014, Mesman 2011).

If healthcare safety and quality are to be more thoroughly understood, their textured nature and multi-dimensional properties drawn out, and a more integrated and programmatic approach provided, it is important that such sociological insights are brought to the fore. The aim of the *22nd Sociology of Health & Illness Monograph* is to further this aspiration by showcasing some exemplary studies. It offers a reflection on the contribution sociology can make and is making to the healthcare quality and safety agenda and raises some critical questions about the future of sociological engagement. How can we understand and explain the social, cultural and lived experiences of quality and safety? What theories, models and concepts are useful in progressing the quality and safety agenda? What is the appropriate balance between a sociology 'of' and a sociology 'for' quality and safety? What distinctly sociological research approaches might be applied to the study of quality and safety? What analytical perspectives might offer novel insights?

Parallel paths?

The first chapter in the collection reviews the emergence of this field and traces its evolution. Waring *et al.* argue that research and practice in quality and safety has progressed along two largely parallel paths. While an orthodox paradigm, dominated by those pursuing medical and safety science, has largely set the agenda in this field, the sociological paradigm has offered a more critical and nuanced understanding of these issues drawing on central disciplinary concerns such as: expertise and knowledge, the professions and healthcare division of labour, deviance and social control, risk, socio-technical innovation, governance and regulation, experiences of health and illness, organisational culture, help-seeking behaviour, professional-patient relationships, power and politics, and bureaucracies and institutions. There is now an accumulated body of sociological knowledge to provide the foundations for systematic engagement with dominant understandings of the problem of healthcare quality and safety and approaches to the management of risk and error and the chapters in this collection signal some fruitful directions of travel.

Organising for safety and quality

The first theme in the Monograph considers organising for quality and safety. Within the orthodox paradigm many see the solution to healthcare quality and safety in the restructuring and reorganisation of healthcare work (e.g. Chang *et al.* 2005, Donaldson 2009, Woloshynowych *et al.* 2005). This rationalist view is founded on the belief that organisational systems can be engineered and that revising formal structures and processes is the key to safer, more effective and efficient service delivery. From a sociological perspective, such assumptions are overly reductionist, and can often result in mechanistic interventions which have unintended negative consequences. For example, Braithwaite *et al.* (2006) found that restructuring large hospitals had deleterious effects – such as confusion and inefficiencies – rather than creating more streamlined systems, and Fulop *et al.* (2005) found that restructuring put people back at least eighteen months in terms of managerial and planning progress. Oxman (2005) and Braithwaite *et al.* (2005) went even further, and questioned the preoccupation with restructuring health systems activities, parodying the efficacy, the relevance and even the sanity of continually applying the structural 'solution' with no obvious benefits. Infante (2006), coming from a different angle, eschewed managerialist-oriented optimism about the possibility of organising for quality and safety, arguing against the very idea that systems are able simply to respond to some form of 'rolled out' improvement activities. For Infante, a 'system' is an abstraction, even a kind of mirage, and progress is infeasible without adequate theorisation at the centre of which lie relationships, power, culture and complexity. As a rich body of sociological research has shown, healthcare work is complex and its organisation challenging. There will always be a human spirit which wants to see complex problems addressed through the application of clear answers and solutions. Unfortunately, it is rare for the world to yield to this kind of simplification. Focusing on 'the structure' or 'governance' or 'organisation' in order to address quality and safety while important, represents a partial view. Politics, culture and relationships – all important constructs in making care safe and improving quality – are overlooked when excessive attention is placed on structural factors.

The governance and coordination of patient safety is thus a significant organisational challenge which remains theoretically and methodologically under-developed. The chapters in this section attempt to address this problem. Freeman *et al.* draw on observational data from four hospital Foundation Trusts to offer insights into the operation of hospital boards in the English NHS. Boards are responsible for ensuring the quality of care and safety of patients under their jurisdiction. Following Hajer and Versteeg (2005), Freeman *et al.* combine elements from the conceptual frameworks of dramaturgy (Goffman 1974) and performativity (Austin 1962) to explore the enacted dimensions of patient safety governance. The chapter is underpinned by the idea that 'reality is mediated through the application of frames', and examines the socio-cultural nature of patient safety as administered by Executive Boards, focusing in particular on the processing and interpretation of performance data. Despite the distance between them, Freeman *et al.* found an unexpected influence from the Executive Board at the 'blunt end' of the hospital on the clinical frontline. Executive Boards can set the scene and through their activities establish a tone for patient safety and quality across the organisation. The Boards in Freeman *et al.*'s study focused attention differently and through this, established different standards and priorities.

Shifting focus, Mackintosh and Sandall drill down into the world of seriously ill patients and through observations and staff interviews examine the frontline organisation of how patients are identified, rescued and resuscitated in medical and maternity settings. Applying Strauss *et al.*'s (1985) classic patient trajectory concept they examine patients' journeys to show how 'rescue work' differed across the two contexts. In maternity services, patients were typically healthy and adverse events few, staff were alert to crises and they mobilised their capacity to be responsive when necessary. In contrast, in the medical wards where patients were older, more infirm and longer-term, it was accepted that rescue was necessary but that sometimes patients would die. The structures and organisational arrangements in these study sites were poorly designed to meet the needs of this patient population and as a consequence, deterioration was much harder to forecast and more difficult to manage. All in all, the complexity of rescue and resuscitation in the medical wards with patients with multiple conditions and co-morbidities was more demanding and difficult than it was in the corresponding maternity settings. In these chosen hospitals, younger maternal patients were effectively being prioritised over complex, older patients.

A central sociological concern is the interaction between the individual and the system of which they are part. This has been a deep preoccupation of sociologists and manifests in diverse ways in the work of many thinkers. Examples are Giddens's (1984) structuration theory, through the ethnomethodology of Garfinkel (1974), to Scott's (1995) work on institutional theory. Aveling *et al.*'s chapter goes to the heart of such debates about the relationship between structure and agency, and focuses on how hospitals address managing individual versus collective accountability for patient safety. They draw on a rich ethnographic database in five hospitals: three in a high income country (UK), and two from low income countries (both in Africa). They reach into the work of two key theorists to render a framework for their study. Following Thompson (1980), they conceptualise healthcare work as a 'problem of many hands' and combine this with Pellegrino's (2004) four principles for organising (there ought to be an organised system; accountability for each health professional; individual competence and character; and systems reinforcement of these) to frame their analysis. In clear echoes of Giddens's (1984) structuration theory, they show empirically that individuals influence the systems of care, while simultaneously being shaped by that system. The existing model of accountability within the orthodox paradigm, which implies that somehow the individual is accountable independently of the system in which he or she acts, is called into question. Systems and individuals are co-constitutive, interdependent, and their relationships are recursive. In other words, people are subject to social forces, and the impact of social forces is mediated by social action.

All of this is not to say that individuals are not responsible agents, and of course they need to be held to account for their actions. But for Aveling *et al.*, systems need to support both individual and communal professionalism and accountability. Simplistic patient safety models which blame individuals or make them individually responsible for group activities should thus be rejected. Aveling *et al.*'s analysis lays the foundation for more sophisticated models of accountability than allowed by the narrowly instrumental frameworks which dominate the orthodox paradigm.

Technologies and practices of quality and safety

The second theme in the collection centres on technologies and practices of quality and safety. Healthcare is a technologically intensive and dynamic environment, with new interventions emerging regularly. These range from the most sophisticated (and expensive) scanner or item of surgical equipment, through new medications and treatments, to everyday 'mundane' technologies such as the patient record and care-plan. All have a bearing on the social organisation of the work and hence healthcare quality and safety. In addition, a range of infrastructural technologies are used in healthcare to organise and support work activity, and many quality improvement initiatives and safety interventions hinge on the introduction of artefacts or tools to bring about behavioural change in the workplace. Examples include surgical checklists, patient status at a glance whiteboards (one of the foundation modules of the UK National Health Service Institute for Innovation and Improvement Productive Ward series) and early warning scores (see McIntosh and Sandall this volume). Yet while the orthodox approach to patient safety has developed and promoted numerous technological solutions to quality and safety problems, it has been rather less adept at theorising the operation of the technology itself and how it is anticipated to have its effects in different contexts. It is also the case that the implementation (or not) of such technologies often rests on a poor understanding of the fundamental nature of the work processes they propose to modify (Allen, in press). The effect of this double neglect is that all too often interventions are routinely imported into healthcare from other fields – such as aviation or manufacturing – with little consideration of sector differences, and progress straight to implementation with scant attention to problem diagnosis as a precursor to intervention selection and/or development. This, as Dixon-Woods (2013) has observed, is equivalent to by-passing the laboratory and pre-clinical and pharmacokinetic stages of drug development.

There is considerable scope for sociologists to contribute to this technology-practice agenda. Under the influence of scholarship in Science and Technology Studies, the sociology of healthcare work (Hughes 1984, Strauss *et al.* 1985) has developed to generate a rich vein of empirical research on healthcare practices and, in particular, the effects of new technologies and their interaction with the social organisation of practice in the workplace. Insights from the sociology of healthcare work prompt critical questions about the intersection of new technologies with extant socio-technical arrangements. Marc Berg has been a leading contributor to this field offering insights into the impact of medical records (Berg 1996), protocols (Berg 1997c) and related health information technologies (Berg 1999) on healthcare work. A fundamental tenet of this scholarship is that formal tools can transform workplaces in important ways (Berg 1997a), but that their generative power can neither be attributed to the tool nor its users; rather it arises instead from their inter-relationship in action. Technologies embody diverse assumptions or scripts and are structured in different ways that are consequential for their impact on the organisation of work. Berg (1999) argues that there is a need to understand this relationship, not least because tools do not slip into some predefined space in the workplace; getting a tool to function as intended requires sensitivity to the work setting (see for example, Berg 1997b, Brown and Webster 2004, Webster 2002). All too often resistance to new technologies in healthcare is interpreted by quality and safety advocates as symptomatic of wider tensions between healthcare professionals or managers or seen as an implementation problem in need of culture management or better leadership. It may also be the case, however, that technologies are genuinely a poor fit with professional practice (Allen 2014, in press; Macintosh *et al.* 2014).

Szymczak's chapter speaks to these concerns. It focuses on the limitations of interventions drawn from aviation designed to encourage clinicians to come forward in the face of known threats to patient safety. These include reporting errors and near misses, blowing the whistle on the poor conduct of colleagues (Jones and Kelly 2014) and encouraging clinicians to raise concerns before harm reaches the patient (Lindsay *et al.* 2012). Szymczak examines an intervention designed to encourage clinicians to 'speak up' and argues that, despite the efforts of patient safety advocates, speaking up remains difficult. Orthodox approaches to this problem focus on individual-cognitive or organisational factors. Demonstrating the value of taking a distinctly sociological approach to a safety problem, Szymczak deploys Collins's (2004) theory of interaction ritual chains to explore clinicians' accounts of speaking up in the context of potential breaches to hospital acquired infections in a US hospital. Three mediating factors are identified that influence the decision to speak up. First, Collins (2004) suggests that successful interaction rituals require participants to have a shared focus of attention. Szymczak observes, however, that despite healthcare providers being co-present in their work, they are not all necessarily focused on the same thing and raising concerns in such a context could have a potentially inflammatory and disruptive effect on the ongoing flow of action. Second, speaking up is interactionally path dependent, that is, decisions to speak up or not are mediated by past experiences as well as those that are anticipated in the future. The data presented here reveal participants to be acutely sensitive to their relationships with other healthcare professionals. Third, speaking up is influenced by the presence of an audience. Collins argues that interaction rituals are facilitated when there is a barrier to outsiders. Much healthcare work takes place in the presence of an audience – such as family members – and clinicians indicated that this was a further factor shaping their decision to speak up. What emerges from the chapter, then, is recognition that in a given moment, the decision to speak up or remain silent, is highly context dependent and embedded in the interaction rituals that shape everyday work. Szymczak argues that teaching scripted communication, as is the custom in aviation, can only have a limited impact on practice; it is not the words that clinicians struggle to find, it is the *place* and *way* to integrate them into the ongoing flow of action that is the issue.

A further insight offered by sociological studies of healthcare work is that many quality and safety interventions do not take into account the invisible daily practices through which healthcare quality is achieved (Allen 2014, Mesman 2011). Grant *et al.*'s chapter contributes further to these sociological insights. Applying Strauss *et al.*'s (1985) scholarship on 'articulation work' and drawing on extensive ethnographic research in NHS Scotland and NHS England they examine the invisible work of general practice team members in the achievement of repeat prescribing. Repeat prescriptions are medications for long-term use, typically for chronic conditions, and are issued without a consultation between the patient and prescriber. This is a high volume process in which risk and vulnerability are distributed across time and space, in a context in which medications management is a significant cause of adverse events. While clinicians are often the primary object of quality and safety interventions, Grant *et al.* illuminate the contribution of non-clinical staff – in this case GP receptionists – and make an important addition to the growing literature on this hitherto relatively neglected group (Arber and Sawyer 1985, Copeman and van Zwanenberg 1988, Swinglehurst *et al.* 2011). Viewed through the lens of articulation work, the study reveals the central role of the informal, invisible practices of receptionists, with informal cross-hierarchical communication often more effective than formal organisational structures. The chapter adds further weight to an emerging body of sociologically informed research which underscores the imperfect and contingent character of healthcare work and its attendant risks. Rules, guidelines and protocols have self-evident limitations in ensuring healthcare quality and safety in such circumstances, with quality and safety being dependent to a considerable extent on the informal resources of resilience and practical wisdom employed by local teams (Hollnagel *et al.* 2013, Wears *et al.* 2015).

Experiences, and contribution to quality and safety

The final theme focuses on experiences of quality and safety. It is concerned with the meaning of quality and safety for patients, professionals, managers and policymakers, and the implications this has for the relationships between different actors as they negotiate quality and safety in the clinical encounter or secure quality improvement across stakeholder boundaries. Prior work on patient safety has focused mainly on systems and professionals, but there is an emerging interest in patients' contributions to their own safety. Since 2004, Patients for Patient Safety (PFPS) has emphasised the role patients and consumers can play in efforts to improve the quality and safety of healthcare around the world. PFPS works with a global network of patients, consumers, caregivers, and consumer organisations to support patient involvement in patient safety programmes, both within countries and in the global programmes of the WHO Patient Safety. The ultimate purpose is to improve safety in all healthcare settings throughout the world by involving service users and patients as partners, and through the development of patient-focused empowerment tools to support help seeking. Patients and their families see things that busy healthcare workers often do not.

The voice of patients and families who have suffered preventable medical injury is a powerful motivational force for healthcare providers across the globe. However, patients have much more to offer than as the victims of tragic medical errors. Important as that perspective is, a victim orientation does not position service users as partners working with healthcare providers to prevent harm. Indeed, the perception that patients and their families are helpless or antagonistic victims has served to distance service users from playing meaningful roles in the development and implementation of patient safety work in the past and has generated fear among some clinicians who would have otherwise engaged with the process (Annandale 1996). At the service delivery level, patients who wish to contribute knowledge gained or lessons learned have often found few effective pathways for doing so (Snow et al. 2013). Particularly after healthcare accidents occur, a 'wall of silence' may descend and productive interaction may cease. When patients and families register concerns, their actions often are perceived as adversarial threats or unscientific anecdotes that lack evidence, rather than potential knowledge contributions. Although there are notable exceptions, at the policymaking level user participation tends to be marginalised too, often by well meaning leaders who assume patients and families are unable to appreciate the complexity of healthcare (Iedema et al. 2008, 2011). Such an approach fails to take into account that many users offer the richest resource of information related to medical errors as many have witnessed every detail of system failures from the beginning to end.

There is some evidence that patients report suspected adverse events earlier than professionals, suggesting that increased patient involvement has the potential to reduce delay in the identification and treatment of problems (Egberts et al. 1996, Coulter and Ellins 2006). However, strategies to improve patient safety have so far mainly focused on changing the organisation of delivery and provider behaviour and paid limited attention to the ways in which patients already contribute to their own safety (Vincent and Coulter 2002). A handful of initiatives, mainly from the USA, have been designed to empower patients and relatives to escalate care themselves. These include 'SBAR for patients' which develops the application of structured communication tools developed for use between health professionals (Denham 2008), 'family-activated paediatric Rapid Response Systems' (Ray et al. 2009, Entwistle et al. 2005) and the 'Speak up for patient safety' campaign in the USA.

While the scope for involvement is considerable, there is limited understanding of the potential for patients and relatives to contribute to their own safety, the contextual circumstances that moderate acceptability and the effectiveness of various interventions which might promote this, and potential unintended consequences (Davis et al. 2007). For example, patients in some settings were reluctant to challenge professionals, and were further discouraged from doing so if their concerns were not heard or attended to (Rainey et al. 2013), and even when service users did speak up, they found that staff did not take their concerns seriously (Rance et al. 2013). Furthermore, assertions about the benefit of patient involvement have been based on experiences of chronic disease management, rather than acute episodes of care which may involve life threatening events, and thus assume a level of agency that does not exist in all cases (Peat et al. 2010). There has been little research on understanding the organisational context and influences of staff responses to patient concerns (Dixon-Woods et al. 2014).

Two chapters in this Monograph explore these issues in the under researched settings of primary care and mental health. Sanders et al. draw on Weick's (1995) concept of sensemaking, and explore the ways in which patients make sense of their experiences of primary medical care and how that conditions their conceptualisation of safety. In qualitative interviews with primary care patients in England, patients reported being proactive in taking action to protect themselves from potential harm within the context of the routinised and predictable nature of the primary medical care consultation. The authors argue that this contrasts with previous research that highlights the relative passivity of patients in acute hospital settings. Patients had to balance different dimensions of safety and weigh them against other concerns and social imperatives. Safety, for patients, was not necessarily always their top priority, and their preferences may not always have been considered 'safe' from the perspective of health professionals. Their accounts draw attention to a largely invisible and inaccessible (but taken for granted) safety infrastructure, the importance of trust and psycho-social as well as physical dimensions of safety and the interactions between them, informal strategies for negotiating safety, and the moral dimension of safety. The ability to take a proactive role was dependent on patients' expertise and knowledge accumulated over time, the social distance between doctor and patient, and patients' self-confidence. In consequence, some patients were more able to adopt a questioning, assertive and proactive role than others.

In the mental health context, Brown *et al.* report on findings from in-depth interviews with service-users, professionals, managers and other stakeholders across three mental health-care (psychosis) teams in England, in what is described as a low trust service context. They note that trust has been seen as fundamental for quality healthcare provision and outcomes, enabling action, cooperation and knowledge sharing where these are otherwise problematic. They draw on theoretical understandings of the interlinking of different trust relationships across healthcare settings. They argue that analyses of micro-level mechanisms through which cultures of trust or distrust propagate are vital to sociological studies of quality and safety due to the ways in which trusting relations underpin patient's sharing of information, and the flow of knowledge within healthcare organisations. Describing chains of (dis)trust as a key element of organisational culture, they explain how (dis)trust within one intra-organisational relationship impacts upon other relationships. They explore how knowledge-sharing and care giving are interwoven within these chains of trust or distrust, enhancing and/or inhibiting the instrumental and communicative aspects of quality healthcare.

Both chapters highlight the importance of sensemaking as an analytic lens and of the value of looking at the creation or not of trust in two areas of healthcare where there is a paucity of research.

The sociology of quality and safety: future directions

The empirical chapters in this collection address technologies, practices, experiences and the organisation of quality and safety across a wide range of healthcare contexts. Spanning three continents, from hospital to community, maternity to mental health, they shine a light into the boardrooms, back offices and front-lines of healthcare, offering sociological insights from the perspectives of managers, clinicians and patients. In their review of the field, Waring *et al.* argue that hitherto the sociology of quality and safety has evolved in parallel with the orthodox paradigm with relatively little cross-fertilisation beyond critique. As the sociological corpus matures and critical questions about the prevailing orthodoxy gain wider currency (Swinglehurst 2015), the conditions exist for more constructive engagement. In their chapter, Waring *et al.* identify three dilemmas within the current orthodoxy – concretisation, culture and politics – which they argue would benefit from a sociological perspective. In the second part of this chapter we consider how the chapters in this collection contribute to these concerns and outline potential lines of inquiry.

Concretisation

In contrast to the orthodox view which treats quality and safety as 'things' that can be measured, managed and experienced, the chapters presented here add further weight to the value of a distinctly sociological understanding of quality and safety as emergent processes, mediated through complex networks of actors. As Aveling *et al.*'s chapter observes, healthcare quality and safety are a 'work of many hands' and while their specific concern is with the implications of this insight for accountability, it is also consequential for an understanding of how quality and safety is accomplished and by extension how best it might be supported. There is a growing appreciation that for all the policies, protocols and standards, achieving quality and safety across time and space depends to a considerable extent on practical wisdom which, as Grant *et al.*'s chapter on repeat prescribing has shown, is often invisible to the organisation. While formal processes are important and demand serious attention, efforts to improve quality and safety are destined to fail if these intentions are based on a partial understanding of the work (Allen 2014). There are also very real risks that the introduction of new technologies and structures will unwittingly undermine important sources of organisational resilience. There is a strong tradition of sociological studies of healthcare work (Allen and Pilnick 2006), going back to the classic studies of Hughes (1984) and Strauss *et al.* (1985), and within the field of quality and safety there exists a self-evident niche for programmatic sociological inquiry to better understand the social organisation of contemporary healthcare work as a distributed and cooperative activity. In order to move forward, however, a shift in focus is necessary. While enthusiastic efforts are being made by quality and safety advocates to embed a commitment to quality and safety at all levels of healthcare organisation, as evidenced, for example, by the introduction of the Q Initiative by NHS England and the Health Foundation, sociological studies have for too long been preoccupied by the inner workings of medicine, and to a lesser extent nursing, with relatively little attention given to the work of others within healthcare. Recent research and policy highlights the important contributions of managers, allied health professionals, paramedics, clerical staff, cleaners, caterers and procurement specialists to quality and safety. Such initiatives indicate that future sociological work might consider the diverse range of actors and networks involved in realising improvement, in addition to its longstanding concern with the medical and nursing professions.

A major contribution of Strauss *et al.*'s (1985) study of the social organisation of medical work was the acknowledgement of patients' and families' contribution to healthcare, concerns that were subsequently taken up in their research on chronic disease management (Corbin and Strauss 1988) and more recently in a programme of work on burden of treatment (May *et al.* 2014). As we have seen, there is a growing recognition of the potential for patients and their families to contribute to healthcare quality and safety, but it is less clear how this might be supported given the inequalities of power and expertise which are the hallmark of professional-patient interaction. The contributions by Sanders *et al.* and Brown *et al.* in this monograph call into question to what extent service users' understandings of quality and safety concur with healthcare professionals and how any such discrepancies should be managed. As Sanders *et al.* show, not only is the practice of healthcare quality and safety a distributed and emergent phenomenon, but patient's experience of it is too. There is considerable scope for patient involvement in their own safety but limited understanding of how this potential might be realised, the contextual circumstances that moderate this process, or the various interventions which might promote this. Moreover, if we accept that quality and safety defies concretisation, then this raises the question of how quality and safety are negotiated within the clinical encounter and how quality and safety are balanced and any attendant risks managed. Research into the contribution patients can make to improving the safety of their care is still in its early stages and an area that sociologists are well placed to contribute to.

Culture

While the dominant paradigm has embraced the ostensibly sociological concept of culture, its application can be called into question. On the one hand, culture has been understood as an organisational property that is receptive to change, so that, for example, a blame culture can be turned into a safety-aware culture. On the other hand, it has become a residual category to which policymakers assign all the organisational phenomena outside their control or understanding (Ormond 2003). Sociologists have rightly countered that culture has to be understood as an emergent property of underlying social structures, intrinsically infused with differences, shifting allegiances and variable attitudes, values and predispositions. But if there is a serious intent to engage with policy and practice in this field, emphasising this complexity can only take us so far. Acknowledging culture to be important, but acknowledging the challenges of its operationalisation, Brown *et al.*'s chapter focuses on very specific features of culture – interwoven relations of (dis)trust across organisations – which bear fundamentally on their concerns with the communicative and learning functions of local healthcare services. They argue that: 'Far from capturing all aspects of organisational 'culture', our analysis nevertheless identifies salient processes which help explain important patterns of relationships and meaning across organisations and beyond' (Ormond 2003: 230). Adopting such a lens, they are able to trace chains of trust throughout the organisation and the impact of these on patients. Their enquiry signals the way for more focused sociological work on those specific aspects of organisational culture that are consequential for healthcare quality and safety and their inter-relationships across the diverse contexts, groups and levels within an organisation.

Building on this theme, Freeman *et al.* also point to a potentially fruitful avenue of further research focused on the performative aspects of culture. This moves us away from considerations of culture as a reflection of group sentiments to a conceptualisation in which culture is viewed as a constellation of props, scripts, settings, frames and performances that shape how quality and safety is enacted from board to ward. Understanding culture as practice has potentially important implications for how it might be addressed and taken into account in safeguarding healthcare quality and safety.

These contributions offer a view of culture that avoids treating it as manageable property of an organisation, whilst also showing in very specific ways how cultural characteristics and attributes influence the organisation and delivery of care. Without question, cultures have a significant bearing on quality and safety, and policies are likely to continue calling for culture change as basis for improvement, but sociology has the potential to contribute to the development of more sophisticated understandings of cultures and their role in the advancement of quality and safety.

Politics

The orthodox approach to quality and safety often appears to operate on the assumption that healthcare settings can be rendered benign by appropriate efforts such as team building or transformational leadership; whereas from a sociological perspective, differential resources, interests and ideologies will always be manifest. In their analysis of rescue trajectories, Macintosh *et al.*'s chapter draws attention to how institutional arrangements mitigated 'rescue work' in the care of older people but enforced its prioritisation in the maternity context. There is ample sociological work on social and health inequalities to suppose these institutional sources of disadvantage to be more widespread. Such insights serve as an important cautionary tale for enthusiasts of systems reengineering as a mechanism for service improvement. As Berg and Timmermans (2000) have argued, orders do not emerge out of and thereby replace a pre-existing disorder; rather, with the production of an order, a corresponding disorder comes into being. It is ironic that as the global population ages and the needs of healthcare users become ever more complex, healthcare services are becoming increasingly rationalised, bringing benefits for some and disbenefits for others. In a similar vein, Sanders *et al.* reveal the importance of social capital for patients in negotiating access to services and how those with greater experience of the healthcare system considered themselves to be at an advantage relatively to those who had had less exposure. For all the commitment to patient-centredness within the quality and safety movement it is clear that service users are unequally placed to negotiate this social good.

A further key theme to emerge across the chapters presented here is the relational nature of healthcare quality and safety. Szymczak's examination of interaction chains highlights the importance of professional relationships in influencing participants' decisions to speak up in the face of a potential safety threat and both Brown *et al.* and Sanders *et al.* underline the centrality of provider-patient relationships to users' experiences of quality and safety. Common to both chapters is an emphasis on the importance of 'psychosocial safety' and 'trust', with the technical aspects of quality and safety being largely taken for granted by service users. Indeed, organisational targets and standards were perceived to impinge negatively on their relationships with providers, who they viewed as constrained by performance indicators which reduced contact time and physician discretion. This concern with structure and agency takes centre stage in Aveling *et al.*'s chapter on the relationship between healthcare professionals' moral authority to do the right thing, while recognising that these decisions do not take place outside of healthcare systems. It is also a pivotal concern in Freeman *et al.*'s analysis of how clinical governance is framed and performed by different NHS hospital boards and how such arrangements shape how the governance of quality and safety is enacted within organisations. Such questions about the relationship between social structures and human agency are well-trodden topics within the sociological tradition and an issue that – in the context of quality and safety – would benefit from such expert insights.

The failure to attend to the political structures of healthcare organisation, especially where these are associated with professional power, frames many of the protracted and limited efforts at transformation and improvement. The act of introducing quality improvement often means defining existing practices as imperfect, substandard or problematic; practices that are closely bounded up with professional identities and jurisdictions. As such, resistance to change might not always be seen as recalcitrant groups protecting their jurisdictions or privileges, but also groups seeking to maintain their sense of self or place in the workplace.

Theory and practice

The chapters in this collection signal alternative approaches to the three dilemmas of the orthodox paradigm, and suggest future avenues of empirical sociological inquiry. These centre on the social organisation of work, reconceptualising culture and the politics of structure and agency relationships. But what about theory? Chapters featured here have drawn *inter alia* on established sociological concepts – articulation work, interaction rituals, trajectories, structuration, sensemaking and dramaturgy – all with positive effect. There is also an emerging view that the development and evaluation of interventions to bring about improvements in healthcare quality and safety have been impoverished by a failure to connect with social theory. Against a mounting weight of evidence that an intervention that has been successful in one location will not necessarily deliver the same results elsewhere, there is a growing appreciation of the need to better understand the inter-relationships involved in the content-context-implementation triangle. Theory-driven approaches are widely believed to be central to this aim, necessary to better understand the problem to be addressed, how an intervention has its effects and the modifications and conditions required for successful implementation in different contexts. This has led a number of authors to call for greater collaboration between social scientists and quality improvers (Davidoff *et al.* 2015, Dixon-Woods *et al.* 2011). While there are some nascent efforts to support developers in making their taken-for-granted ethno theories explicit in improvement initiatives (Davidoff *et al.* 2015), attempts to close the theory practice gap have largely involved the importation of existing sociological theories. These are clearly important advances, but if we are to build on the logic of a distinctive sociological conceptualisation of quality and safety, there is also a need to develop new theoretical frameworks to enrich this agenda grounded in the growing corpus of empirical sociological work and/or through close engagement with real life improvement efforts.

Collectively the chapters in this monograph highlight the need for theories and frameworks which support the systematic analysis of the processes that mediate individual agency and structural constraints in producing healthcare quality and safety in which the latter is understood to be both a distributed practice and a negotiated experience. Such mid-range theories are needed which offer new frameworks of understanding and a common language to support research and practice, so that sociology might not only strengthen improvement efforts, but also radically reshape from the inside how the problem of quality and safety is understood, experienced, assessed and studied. A number of the chapters in this collection have sown the seeds of such sociological novelty. Szymczak's use of Collins' concept of interaction rituals offers an alternative understanding of the problem of not speaking up in the context of threats to safety and Aveling *et al.* combine concepts from philosophy (Thompson 1980, 2014) and ethics (Pellegrino 2002, 2004) with structuration theory to reframe individual accountability and moral responsibility in patient safety. We also see potential in theoretical syntheses from within sociology. For example, Grant *et al.* and MacIntosh *et al.* utilise Strauss' classic ideas on articulation work and patient trajectories respectively, but as Allen (2014) as shown, these can be fruitfully combined with more recent theoretical insights from practice-based approaches and in particular actor network theory. Several of the chapters in this collection also contribute to current theoretical developments in the study of governance, which involves new connections between political sociology, interpretative methodologies and social theory (Bevir 2013). In particular, the works of Strauss, Goffman, Foucault and Giddens are invoked in various ways to understand how healthcare quality and safety are organised and governed. This line of analysis contributes to growing interest in the study of governance and social order, not in terms of formal structures, roles or institutions, but rather as situated, embodied and discursive social practices, albeit located within a given historical and structural field. In particular, there is scope to pursue new lines of theoretical synergy by linking different theoretical traditions, such as Strauss' concept of negotiated order with Foucault's work on knowledge/power, to contribute both to the sociological study of healthcare quality and safety, and also new perspectives on governance and relational sociology (Crossley 2012).

Our focus here is on the sociological contribution to healthcare quality and safety, but the management of risk and safety transcends a whole host of organisational locales and sociologists have done much to augment understanding of these issues (Perrow 1984, Vaughan 1997, 1999). As yet, however, there has been no attempt to work programmatically across a diversity of contexts. Healthcare has been deluged with interventions imported from other high risk environments in the expectation that these will confer the same benefits as they have been claimed to have brought elsewhere and sociologists have been quick to critique the naivety of such assumptions. Bosk *et al.* (2009: 445), for example, caution against the overuse of checklists in healthcare:

> The success of checklists in preventing disasters during the takeoff and landing of commercial aircraft is often pointed out. But checklists are also used to track baggage for airlines. On this task, check lists perform less admirably. Handling baggage that comes in different sizes and shapes, involves complex transfers, and is often in poor condition, is a more realistic analogy for the use of checklists in achieving patients' safety than their use on takeoffs and landings. Baggage handling is a task that shares with managing patients a staggering amount of coordination, time-pressured decisionmaking, frustrating delays, and tracking systems for non-standardised raw material that needs to be handled safely.

As the sociology of healthcare quality and safety comes of age, there is not only scope for insight from healthcare to be applied to other organisational contexts but also for more collaborative working between social scientists with expertise in different industries and domains. As Hughes's (1984) classic studies of work have shown, much can be learnt from analysing such commonalities and differences. Evidence syntheses are only recently emerging in the social sciences, but as empirical work on quality and safety accumulates, more needs to be done to advance theories grounded in this cumulative material. It is from such foundations that we have the prospect of advancing a sociology of quality and safety that transcends organisations and institutions.

Acknowledgements

Jane Sandall was supported by the National Institute for Health Research (NIHR) Collaboration for Leadership in Applied Health Research and Care South London at King's College Hospital NHS Foundation Trust. Justin Waring was supported by the National Institute for Health Research (NIHR) Collaboration for Leadership in Applied Health Research and Care East Midlands. The views expressed are those of the author(s) and not necessarily those of the NHS, the NIHR or the Department of Health.

References

Allen, D. (2014) *The Invisible Work of Nurses: Hospitals, Organisation and Healthcare*. London: Routledge.
Allen, D. and Pilnick, A. (eds) (2006) *The Social Organisation of Healthcare Work*. London: Sage.
Annandale, E. (1996) Working on the front-line: risk culture and nursing in the new NHS, *The Sociological Review*, 44, 3, 416–51.

Arber, S. and Sawyer, L. (1985) The role of the receptionist in general practice: A 'dragon behind the desk'?, *Social Science & Medicine*, 20, 9, 911–21.

Austin, J.L. (1962) *How to do Things with Words.* Cambridge, MA: Harvard University Press.

Berg, M. (1996) Practice of reading and writing: the constitutive role of the patient record in medical work, *Sociology of Health & Illness*, 18, 4, 499–524.

Berg, M. (1997a) *Rationalizing Medical Work: Decision-support Techniques and Medical Practices.* Cambridge: Cambridge University Press.

Berg, M. (1997b) On distribution, drift and the electronic medical record: some tools for a sociology of the formal. J Hughes *et al.* (eds) Proceedings of the Fifth European Conference on Computer Supported Cooperative Work, 141–56. The Netherlands: Kluwer Academic Publishers.

Berg, M. (1997c) Problems and promises of the protocol, *Social Science and Medicine*, 44, 8, 1081–8.

Berg, M. (1999) Accumulating and coordinating: occasions for information technologies in medical work, *Computer Supported Cooperative Work*, 8, 4, 373–401.

Berg, M. and Timmermans, S. (2000) Orders and their others: on the constitution of universalities in medical work, *Configurations*, 8, 1, 31–61.

Bevir, M. (2013) *A Theory of Governance.* Berkeley, VA: University of California Press.

Bosk, C. (1979) *Forgive and Remember: Managing Error: The Culture of Safety on the Shop Floor.* Princeton, NJ: Institute for Advanced Study.

Bosk, C., Dixon-Woods, M., Goeschel, C.A., Pronovost, P., *et al.* (2009) Reality check for checklists, *The Lancet*, 374, 9688, 444–5.

Braithwaite, J., Westbrook, J. and Iedema, R. (2005) Restructuring as gratification, *Journal of the Royal Society of Medicine*, 98, 12, 542–4.

Braithwaite, J., Westbrook, M.T., Hindle, D., Iedema, R.A., *et al.* (2006) Does restructuring hospitals result in greater efficiency – an empirical test using diachronic data, *Health Services Management Research*, 19, 1, 1–12.

Braithwaite, J., Matsuyama, Y., Mannion, R., Johnson, J., *et al.* (2015) *Healthcare Reform, Quality and Safety: Perspectives, Participants, Partnerships and Prospects in 30 Countries.* Farnham: Ashgate.

Brown, N. and Webster, A. (2004) *New Medical Technologies and Society.* Cambridge: Polity Press.

Chang, A., Schyve, P.M., Croteau, R.J., O'Leary, D.S., *et al.* (2005) The JCAHO patient safety event taxonomy: a standardised terminology and classification schema for near misses and adverse events, *International Journal for Quality in Healthcare*, 17, 1, 95–105.

Collins, R. (2004) *Interaction Ritual Chains.* Princeton, NJ: Princeton University Press.

Copeman, J. and van Zwanenberg, T. (1988) Practice receptionists: poorly paid and taken for granted?, *Journal of the Royal College of General Practitioners*, 38, 1, 14–6.

Corbin, J. and Strauss, A. (1988) *Unending Work and Care: Managing Chronic Illness at Home.* San Francisco CA: Jossey Bass.

Coulter, A. and Ellis, J. (2006) *Patient-focused Interventions: A Review of the Evidence.* London: Picker Institute/Health Foundation.

Crossley, N. (2012) *Towards Relational Sociology.* London: Routledge.

Davidoff, F., Dixon-Woods, M., Leviton, L., Michie, S., *et al.* (2015) Demystifying theory and its use in improvement, *BMJ Quality and Safety*, 24, 3, 228–38.

Davis, R.E., Jacklin, R., Sevdalis, N., Vincent, C., *et al.* (2007) Patient involvement in patient safety: what factors influence patient participation and engagement?, *Health Expectations*, 10, 3, 259–67.

Denham, C.R. (2008) SBAR for patients, *Journal of Patient Safety*, 4, 1, 38–48.

Dingwall, R. and Allen, D. (2001) The implications of healthcare reforms for the profession of nursing, *Nursing Inquiry*, 8, 2, 64–74.

Dixon-Woods, M. (2010) Why is patient safety so hard? A selective review of ethnographic studies, *Journal of Health Services Research and Policy*, 15, 1, 1–16.

Dixon-Woods, M. (2013) The problem of context in quality improvement. In *Perspectives on Context: A Selection of Essays Considering the Role of Context in Successful Quality Improvement.* London: The Health Foundation.

Dixon-Woods, M., Bosk, C.L., Aveling, E.L., Goeschel, C.A., *et al.* (2011) Explaining Michigan: developing an ex post theory of a quality improvement program, *The Milbank Quarterly*, 89, 2, 167–205.

Dixon-Woods, M., Baker, R., Charles, K., Dawson, J., *et al.* (2014) Culture and behaviour in the English National Health Service: overview of lessons from a large multimethod study, *BMJ Quality & Safety*, 23, 2, 106–15.

Donaldson, L. (2009) An international language for patient safety: global progress in patient safety requires classification of key concepts, *International Journal for Quality in Healthcare*, 21, 1, 1.

Egberts, T.C.G., Smulders, M., de Koning, F.H.P., Meyboom, R.H.B., *et al.* (1996) 'Can adverse drug reactions be detected earlier? A comparison of reports by patients and professionals', *BMJ*, 313, 7056, 530–1.

Entwistle, V., McCaughan, D., Watt, I.S., Hall, J., *et al.* (2010) Speaking up about safety concerns: multi-setting qualitative study of patients' views and experiences, *BMJ Quality & Safety*, 19, 6, 1–7.

Entwistle, V.A., Michelle, M.M. and Brennan, T.A. (2005) Advising patients about patient safety: current initiatives risk shifting responsibility, *Joint Commission Journal on Quality and Patient Safety*, 31, 9, 483–94.

Fox, N. (1999) Postmodern reflections on "risk", "hazards" and life choices. In Lupton, D. (ed.) *Risk and Sociocultural Theory.* Cambridge: Cambridge University Press.

Fulop, N., Protopsaltis, G., King, A., Allen, P., *et al.* (2005) Changing organisations: a study of the context and processes of mergers of healthcare providers in England, *Social Science and Medicine*, 60, 1, 119–30.

Garfinkel, H. (1974) The origins of the term ethnomethodology. In Turner, R. (ed.) *Ethnomethodology.* Harmondsworth: Penguin.

Giddens, A. (1984) *The Constitution of Society: Outline of the Theory of Structuration.* Cambridge: Polity Press.

Goffman, E. (1974) *Frame Analysis. An Essay on the Organisation of Experience.* Boston, MA: Northeastern University Press.

Hajer, M. and Versteeg, W. (2005) Performing governance through networks, *European Political Science*, 4, 340–7.

Hall, J., Peat, M., Birks, Y. and Golder, S., on behalf of PIPS Group (2010) Effectiveness of interventions designed to promote patient involvement to enhance safety: a systematic review, *Quality Saf Healthcare*, Oct, 19, 5, e10.

Hollnagel, E., Braithwaite, J. and Wears, R.L. (eds) (2013) *Resilient Healthcare.* Farnham: Ashgate.

Hughes, E.C. (1984) *The Sociological Eye.* New Brunswick, NJ: Transaction Books.

Iedema, R., Long, D., Carroll, K., Stenglin, M., *et al.* (2006) Corridor work: how luminal spaces becomes a resource for handling complexities of multidisciplinary healthcare, Pacific Researchers in Organisational Studies 11th Colloquium, 238–47. Available at http://search.informit.com.au/documentSummary;dn=305691933675194;res=IELBUS (accessed 27 July 2015).

Iedema, R., Sorensen, R., Manias, E., Tuckett, A., *et al.* (2008) Patients' and family members' experiences of open disclosure following adverse events, *International Journal for Quality in Healthcare*, 20, 6, 421–32.

Iedema, R., Allen, S., Britton, K., Piper, D., *et al.* (2011) Patients' and family members' views on how clinicians enact and how they should enact incident disclosure: the "100 patient stories" qualitative study, *BMJ*, 343: d4423.

Illich, I. (1976) *Medical Nemesis: The Exploration of Health.* New York: Pantheon Books.

Infante, C. (2006) Bridging the "system's" gap between interprofessional care and patient safety: sociological insights, *Journal of Interprofessional Care*, 20, 5, 517–25.

Jensen, C.B. (2008) Sociology, systems and (patient) safety; knowledge translations in healthcare policy, *Sociology of Health & Illness*, 30, 2, 309–24.

Jones, A. and Kelly, D. (2014) Whistle-blowing and workplace culture in older peoples' care: qualitative insights from the healthcare and social care workforce, *Sociology of Health & Illness*, 36, 7, 986–1002.

Lindsay, P., Sandall, J. and Humphrey, C. (2012) The social dimensions of safety incident reporting in maternity care: The influence of working relationships and group processes, *Social Science & Medicine*, 75, 10, 1793–9.

Mackintosh, N. and Sandall, J. (2010) Overcoming gendered and professional hierarchies in order to facilitate escalation of care in emergency situations: the role of standardised communication protocols, *Social Science & Medicine*, 71, 9, 1683–6.

Macrae, C. (2014) *Close Calls: Managing Risk and Resilience in Airline Flight Safety.* Basingstoke: Palgrave Macmillan.

Magee, M. and Askham, J. (2008) *Women's Views about Safety in Maternity Care: A Qualitative Study.* London: The King's Fund/Picker Institute Maternity Services Inquiry.

May, C., Eton, D.T., Boehmer, K., Gallacher, K., *et al.* (2014) Rethinking the patient: using burden of treatment theory to understand the changing dynamics of illness, *BMC Health Services Research*, 14, 281.

Mesman, J. (2011) *Uncertainty in Medical Innovation: Experienced Pioneers in Neonatal Care.* Basingstoke: Palgrave Macmillan.

Mol, A. (2008) *Health and the Problem of Patient Choice.* New York: Routledge.

Ormond, S. (2003) Organisational culture in health service policy and research: 'third way political fad or policy development?, *Policy and Politics*, 31, 2, 227–37.

Oxman, A.D., Sackett, D.L., Chalmers, I., Prescott, T.E., *et al.* (2005) A surrealistic mega-analysis of redisorganisation theories, *Journal of the Royal Society of Medicine*, 98, 12, 563–8.

Peat, M., Entwistle, V., Hall, J., Birks, Y., *et al.* (2010) Scoping review and approach to appraisal of interventions intended to involve patients in patient safety, *Journal of Health Services Research & Policy*, 15, 1, 17–25.

Pellegrino, E.D. (2002) Professionalism, profession and the virtues of the good physician, *Mt Sinai Journal of Medicine*, 69, 6, 378–84.

Pellegrino, E.D. (2004) *Prevention of medical error: Where professional and organisational ethics meet. Accountability: Patient Safety and Policy Reform.* Washington, DC: Georgetown University Press.

Perrow, C. (1984) *Normal Accidents: Living with High-Risk Technologies.* Princeton, NJ: Princeton University Press.

Rainey, H., Sandall, J., Ehrich, K., Mackintosh, N., *et al.* (2013) The role of patients and their relatives in 'speaking up' about their own safety – a qualitative study of acute illness, *Health Expectations*, 18, 3, 392–405.

Rance, S., McCourt, C., Rayment, J., Mackintosh, N., *et al.* (2013) Women's safety alerts in maternity care: is speaking up enough?, *BMJ Quality and Safety*, 22, 4, 348–55.

Ray, E.M., Smith, R., Massie, S., Erickson, J., *et al.* (2009) Family alert: implementing direct family activation of a pediatric rapid response team, *The Joint Commission Journal on Quality and Patient Safety*, 35, 11, 575–80.

Rosenthal, M. (1995) *The Incompetent Doctor.* Buckingham: Open Press University.

Scott, W.R. (1995) *Institutions and Organisations.* Thousand Oaks, CA: Sage.

Snow, R., Humphrey, C. and Sandall, J. (2013) What happens when patients know more than their doctors? Diabetics' experiences of health interactions after patient education: a qualitative patient-led study, *BMJ Open*, 3, 11, e003583.

Strauss, A.L., Fagerhaugh, S., Suczek, B., Wiener, C., *et al.* (1985) *Social Organisation of Medical Work.* Chicago, IL: University of Chicago Press.

Swinglehurst, D. (ed.) (2015) The many meanings of 'quality' in healthcare: interdisciplinary perspectives, *BMC Health Services Research*, 15.

Swinglehurst, D., Greenhalgh, T., Russell, J., Myall, M., *et al.* (2011) Receptionist input to quality and safety in repeat prescribing in UK general practice: ethnographic case study, *British Medical Journal*, 343, d6788.

Thompson, D.F. (1980) Moral responsibility of public officials: the problem of many hands, *The American Political Science Review*, 74, 4, 905–16.

Thompson, D.F. (2014) Responsibility for failures of government: the problem of many hands, *American Review of Public Administration*, 44, 3, 259–73.

Timmermans, S. and Berg, M. (1997) Standardization in action: achieving local universality through medical protocols, *Social Studies of Science*, 27, 2, 273–305.

Vaughan, D. (1997) *The Challenger Launch Decision: Risky Technology, Culture and Deviance at NASA.* Chicago, IL: University of Chicago Press.

Vaughan, D. (1999) The dark side of organisations: mistake, misconduct, and disaster, *Annual Review of Sociology*, 25, 271–305.

Vincent, C.A. and Coulter, A. (2002) Patient safety: what about the patient?, *Quality and Safety in Healthcare*, 11, 1, 76–80.

Waring, J. (2005) Beyond blame: cultural barriers to medical incident reporting, *Social Science and Medicine*, 60, 9, 1927–35.

Waring, J. (2013) What Safety–II might learn from the socio-cultural critique of safety–I. In Hollnagel, E., Braithwaite, J. and Wears, R. (eds) *Resilient Healthcare.* London: Ashgate.

Wears, R.L., Hollnagel, E. and Braithwaite, J. (2015) *Resilient Healthcare, Volume 2: The Resilience of Everyday Clinical Work.* Farnham: Ashgate.

Webster, A. (2002) Innovative health technologies and the social: redefining health, medicine and the body, *Current Sociology*, 50, 3, 443–57.

Weick, K.E. (1995) *Sensemaking in Organisations.* Thousand Oaks, CA: Sage.

Woloshynowych, M., Rogers, S., Taylor-Adams, S. and Vincent, C. (2005) The investigation and analysis of critical incidents and adverse events in healthcare, *Health Technology Assessment*, 9, 19, 1 –143.

World Health Organisation (WHO) (2002) Quality of care: patient safety Resolution WHA55.18. Available at http://www.who.int/patientsafety/about/wha_resolution/en/ (accessed 7 November 2015).

2

Healthcare quality and safety: a review of policy, practice and research

Justin Waring, Davina Allen, Jeffrey Braithwaite and Jane Sandall

Introduction

While concerns about the quality and safety of patient care might be traced back to Hippocrates and his famous admonition, 'first, do no harm', the current policy momentum is a relatively recent phenomena. It was not until the early 1990s that clinical risk and patient safety were seriously recognised as service-level problems, and only in the early 2000s that they became major international priorities. Even then, the problems of quality and safety were often precipitated by major service scandals that vacillated between blaming negligent or criminal professionals, such as Shipman (Smith 2005), or pointing to the failings of the wider health system, such as with Mid-Staffordshire (Francis 2013). Throughout much of the history of modern healthcare, the problems of quality and safety have remained the responsibility of the healthcare professions based upon their claims to expert knowledge, clinical autonomy and self-regulation (Freidson 1970). More recently, however, there has been a growing recognition that efforts to improve quality and safety must also take into account the wider organisation and systems of care.

Since the 1990s, research and practice in healthcare quality and safety has followed two largely parallel paths. On the one hand, the field has been dominated by disciplines such as medical science, social psychology, human factors and safety science, which together have framed how quality and safety is understood, how it should be measured and analysed, and the interventions through which it might be addressed. This has generated significant advances in our understanding of the relationship between the quality of clinical practice and the wider clinical environment and thus how quality might be promoted and risk-avoided. On the other hand, healthcare quality and safety is a longstanding, albeit often implicit, theme in the sociology of health and illness, cutting across a range of classic concerns, including expertise and knowledge; the professions, division of labour and social organisation of healthcare work; deviance and social control; risk; socio-technical innovation; governance and regulation; experiences of health and illness; and organisational culture. More recently, these diverse areas of scholarship have given rise to a new corpus of sociologically informed work with a more explicit quality and safety focus, which offers additional, complementary, and at times critical insights on the problems of quality and safety. There is an emerging consensus that in order to lay down the theoretical, methodological and empirical foundations necessary to advance the study of quality and safety, a more inclusive and multidisciplinary

The Sociology of Healthcare Safety and Quality, First Edition. Edited by Davina Allen, Jeffrey Braithwaite, Jane Sandall and Justin Waring. Chapters © 2016 The Authors. Book Compilation © 2016 Foundation for the Sociology of Health & Illness/Blackwell Publishing Ltd.

approach is required, with some making the case for a new science of improvement (Marshall *et al.* 2013). Thus while social psychology, ergonomics and human factors have done much to advance understanding of the sources of quality and safety within the clinical micro system and work environment, sociology can build on this perspective to furnish insights into the cultural, socio-technical, political and institutional forces that influence care quality. Moreover, sociological insights can also contribute to progressing the aspiration to develop quality and safety improvements that span organisational units or operate at the level of the wider care system. In this study we review the evolution of policy, practice and research in healthcare quality and safety, tracing points of divergence and convergence, and consider the possibilities and implications of greater integration of sociology with the orthodox paradigm.

The emergence of healthcare quality and safety as a social problem

Travaglia (2009) discerns that healthcare quality and safety has passed through several phases or waves of interest (see also Bulger 1973, Cassirer and Anderson 2004, Small and Barach 2002). In the first wave, attention to quality and safety was not concerned with sophisticated technology or complex multi-disciplinary care; it was more a case of the earliest proto-doctors, usually with limited knowledge of disease or human biology, doing what they could for patients in the circumstances in which they found themselves. Throughout this long early history of healthcare, responsibility for quality and safety largely rested with the physician or care-giver. This wave lasted for millennia, through ancient epochs and across the Middle Ages into modern times.

By the nineteenth and early twentieth century, a second wave of interest in quality and safety began to surface. This 'enlightened' period reflected wider developments in the emergence of modern medicine, including significant advances in bio-medical sciences, new techniques, diagnostic tests and imaging capabilities; the expansion of university education; the industrialisation of healthcare; and professionalisation processes (Larson 2013). In the mid-nineteenth century, for example, Ignaz Semmelweis dramatically reduced the rate of infection in his Viennese hospital when he ordered all medical students to wash their hands with chlorinated water before maternal deliveries (Porter 1997, Raju 1999). In the early twentieth century the US physician Ernest Codman called upon doctors to follow the progress of every patient and analyse the causes of any poor outcomes (Codman 1917, Sharpe and Faden 1998) from which he created lists of the sources of error (Davis *et al.* 2002). It is interesting to note, however, that many important advances in knowledge and practices were prohibited by the wider politics of professional power, especially where new knowledge might question the autonomy and legitimacy of the emerging medical professions – a theme reinforced by more contemporary studies of medical regulation (Rosenthal 1995). Running alongside these initiatives, and particularly in the US, malpractice suits began to be brought against practitioners who erred (Stetson and Moran 1934).

The third wave of interest in quality and safety dates from around the 1950s until the late 1980s. It runs in tandem with developments in modern medicine, including the explosion of high technology diagnostic and treatment capabilities, advanced procedures, new pharmaceuticals and the emergence of modern disciplines, such as intensive care, emergency and the surgical specialties (Le Fanu 2011). By the 1960s reports were starting to emerge, for instance, about errors and variations in clinical procedures, and by the 1970s there was mounting concern amongst health insurers about the rising costs of litigation and remedial care. It was at this time that Donabedian (2003) established healthcare quality as a new and leading area of health services research and policy, laying the foundations for the current orthodoxy in quality improvement with his ideas about 'systems thinking', 'input-process-outcome' modelling, systematic records reviews and quality improvement strategies.

Despite growing interest in healthcare quality, the day-to-day reality of substandard care and patient harm remained difficult to address and was assumed to be the responsibility of individual clinicians and thus most appropriately managed through professional regulatory procedures (Freidson 1975). In the early 1990s, however, clinical risk and patient safety was increasingly recognised as a 'service-level' problem. This might be seen as a fourth wave of interest where the problems of quality and safety came to the forefront of international policy and were no longer seen as the province of professional jurisdiction. A pivotal moment was the 1991 publication of the Harvard Medical Practice study (Brennan *et al.* 1991, Leape *et al.* 1991). This retrospective case review of over 30,000 randomly selected hospital records in New York State for 1984 found that adverse events occurred in almost 4 per cent of hospitalisations and nearly 28 per cent were due to negligence. Using weighted totals, they estimated that for the 2.6 million patients treated, there were over 98,000 adverse events in this one particular year. Over the next ten years, similar studies of outcome variation, medical error and adverse incidents have been carried out in Australia, Canada, the US and the UK (see Baker *et al.* 2004, Vincent 2006, Vincent *et al.* 2001, Wennberg 1984, Wilson *et al.* 1995). The growing consensus seemed to suggest that around 10 per cent of patients admitted to hospital would experience some type of adverse event that would prolong their care, result in disability or even cause death.

In parallel to this mounting evidence, the problems of quality and safety were catapulted to the forefront of political attention in the 1990s by a succession of major service scandals, which were especially prominent in the UK. These were not the first examples of service failure, with similar serious shortcomings reported in care home and mental health institutions since the 1960s, but from the late 1990s scandals and their associated public inquiries acquired heightened influence in social and political debate (Hughes 2013). Notable UK examples include the inappropriate and murderous activities of individuals like Beverley Allitt, Rodney Ledward, Harold Shipman and more recently, Victorino Chua. In many of these cases, inquiries point to both the criminal intent of rogue clinicians, but also the failings of healthcare and professional systems to appropriately identify and regulate these individuals (e.g. Smith 2005). For example, the Shipman Inquiry was established to investigate the issues surrounding the activities of general practitioner Harold Shipman who was convicted of the murder of 15 of his patients. Not only did the Inquiry conclude he was the most prolific mass murderer in UK history, taking the lives of up to 215 people, but it identified endemic problems in professional regulation, service governance, and a culture of placing professional interests ahead of patient safety (Smith 2005). Reflecting the growing influence of human factors and safety sciences within the field of patient safety, these inquiries have also highlighted failings at the organisational level, such as the cases of Bristol Royal Infirmary, Winterbourne View care home, and Mid-Staffordshire NHS Trust. The Bristol Royal Infirmary Inquiry was one of the most far-reaching reviews of NHS care following the death of 29 babies undergoing paediatric cardiac surgery at Bristol Royal Infirmary between 1984 and 1995. This highlighted significant problems with patient rights, clinical teamwork, communication and whistle-blowing, accountability systems and organisational cultures (Kennedy 2001). It is no coincidence that these reports were published at around the time that the UK patient safety agenda was emerging and helped to frame a wider policy agenda that might have been more difficult if the existing landscape of professional and organisational regulation was not shown to be lacking (Walshe 2003). Looking beyond the UK, similar high profile scandals have called into question the standards of clinical care, even at those centres of excellence so often praised for their quality. For example, in 2004 the inappropriate injection of Chlorhexidine (an antiseptic) led to the death of Mary L. McClinton at the world famous Virginia Mason hospital. Interestingly, the hospital not only thoroughly investigated this incident – identifying confusion in the storage and preparation of medicines and materials – but used the incident as an opportunity to promote learning and culture change within their organisation.

The growing influence of these inquiries in public discourse has led Stanley and Manthorpe (2004) to suggest that we are now witnessing the 'Age of the Inquiry'; whilst Hindle *et al.* (2006) concluded from their review of eight inquiries in six different countries, that these reports have begun to sound homogenous even where differing predisposing factors are identified. Nevertheless, scandals and inquiries continue to feature in public debate and policy-making, suggesting the recent plethora of quality and safety interventions has not been unequivocally successful and, as Hughes (2013) has observed, that past and present inquiries create regulatory mechanisms which then shape the environments with which future inquiries must contend. This is exemplified by the public inquiry into patient deaths at the Mid-Staffordshire NHS Trust, which showed how substandard care could become easily normalised within the organisational routines and culture of care services, especially if these services were under-resourced and preoccupied with meeting external targets and regulatory requirements over and above the day-to-day responsibilities for dignified patient care (Francis 2013). These past and recent scandals unearth familiar sociological issues around the construction of social problems (Spector and Kituse 2009), moral panics (Cohen 2002), professional dominance (Freidson 1975), the caring division of labour (Allen 2013b), rationing (Hughes and Light 2002), organisational complexity (Braithwaite *et al.* 2013, Perrow 1984), regulatory burden (Power 1997) and cultural issues for staff reporting concerns about colleagues (Ehrich 2006, Jones and Kelly 2014, Lindsay *et al.* 2012), all of which consistently fail to be addressed in mainstream patient safety research and policy.

The contemporary wave of quality and safety research is also associated with specific developments in policy, theory and practice. The publication of landmark reports at the turn of the Century, such as *To Err is Human* (Institute of Medicine 1999), *An Organization with a Memory* (Donaldson 2000) and *Crossing the Quality Chasm* (Institute of Medicine 2001), powerfully demonstrated that safety remained a key service problem, that progress had been painfully slow, and that new ideas were needed to engender future improvements. Drawing on theory and research within social psychology, human factors and safety science, the renewed patient safety movement argued that threats to patient safety rarely stem from individual error, professional incompetence or even negligence, but rather are enabled, conditioned or exacerbated by 'latent' factors located within the wider organisation of clinical practice and patient care. This new line of thinking drew attention to the influence of non-clinical skills, team competencies, and organisational cultures, acknowledging that individualised training and packaged responses were insufficient and that organisational systems or cultures should be modified to enhance the safety of clinical teams. Although at first glance this seems to embrace a more sociological approach, in practice, much of this work fell short of a deep appreciation of social theory and methods, evidenced in the widespread application, but impoverished understanding, of fundamental concepts such as 'culture' and 'system' (Waring 2013).

In this later period, health systems and organisations across the developed world began to introduce specialist agencies devoted to improving quality and safety, such as the National Patient Safety Agency in Britain (2001), the Agency for Healthcare Research and Quality in the USA (1999), and the Australian Council on Safety and Quality in Health Care (2000). All of these share common aspirations for diffusing safety knowledge and tools, measuring harm systematically, introducing next generation policies, coordinating training, and supporting the implementation of improvement initiatives. In concert with these state-sponsored agencies, a range of other foundations, trusts and private bodies, identified a niche they too could occupy in supporting the implementation of improvement strategies, such as the Institute of Healthcare Improvement in the US, the Health Foundation in the UK, the Vinnvård group in Sweden, as well as numerous specialist consulting companies.

Healthcare quality and safety clearly have deep historical antecedents, but it is over the last three decades that the major developments in research, practice and policy have been made. There has been a concomitant growth in sociological work on these issues, but for the most part, this has happened outside of the dominant paradigm, producing divergent understandings of the challenges of quality and safety and how these should be addressed. In the next section, we trace some of these parallel paths.

Understanding quality and safety: parallel perspectives

The orthodox paradigm

The contemporary wave of interest in quality and safety has been predominantly framed by concepts and theories found within medical science, social psychology, ergonomics, human factors and resilience engineering. Rather than seeing errors as the result of individual mistake or failure, which tends towards blaming and encouraging secrecy, the prevailing view is that individual or group performance is conditioned by a variety of upstream factors located in the wider system of care, such as the quality of teamwork or communication, the allocation of tasks, workload scheduling, equipment and resource management, and broader service cultures (Reason 2000). From this perspective, safety research examines the relationships between 'active errors' (cognition errors, slips and trips, or behavioural mistakes) and 'latent' factors (stress, design or team dynamics) located within the wider work setting.

As well as understanding clinical risk in terms of active and latent factors, this approach has popularised linear models of cause-and-effect, as exemplified by the Swiss cheese model.[1] Aligned with this distinctive framing of quality and safety, a range of technologies have been developed to inform how clinical risk and patient harm might be identified (incident reporting, failure mode effect analysis), measured and analysed (root cause analysis, process mapping) and ameliorated (plan-do-act-study-act, structured communication tools, care bundles and similar non-clinical interventions) (Vincent 2006).

The medical profession has played an important role in discrediting, slowly accepting and then promoting quality and safety as policy and practice priorities. Whereas once the quality and safety agenda was seen as challenging traditional customs around self-regulation, it has now become a prominent feature of medical education, revalidation, and professional development. The change in attitude has, arguably, been driven by certain segments of the profession, such as anaesthetics, obstetrics and paediatrics, which experience heightened social and legal pressures in the wake of safety breaches. Professional leaders, such as Don Berwick in the US and Sir Liam Donaldson, the former Chief Medical Office for England, have played a prominent role in advancing the issue of patient safety. This has led to a convergence of medical science and human factors perspectives, precipitating the development of quality and safety improvement along a very particular trajectory. It can be seen, for example, that the 'cause-and-effect' logic of patient safety parallels a similar operating logic within clinical care, which says first, secure a diagnosis, and then treat the patient in line with assembled evidence or derived consensus. There is also a sense in which this model of thinking underscores the promotion of 'improvement' as a science (Marshall *et al.* 2013), affording a level of legitimacy to what might otherwise be regarded as a low status pursuit within the profession. This apparent convergence between medical and safety science might also reflect the ambitions of the medical profession to control this emerging field as a means of maintaining self-regulation, rather than control being externally imposed (Waring 2007). Indeed, a large proportion of developments in the patient safety agenda have focused on medicine, with nursing and other healthcare professions featuring less significantly. Nurses, for example, possess considerable organisational and service practice knowledge and are often responsible for leading and managing quality in day-to-day service delivery but have not been prominent at a policy or strategic level (Allen 2009, 2014).

This dominant paradigm has made important contributions to public, professional and policy understandings of healthcare quality and safety. It has moved analytical attention away from the negligent or malicious clinician to demonstrate that wider factors such as task design, communication patterns, teamwork, the availability of resources, time pressures and work stresses, and the broader configuration of work all impact upon the quality of care through conditioning and shaping individual and group performance. In addition, it has generated improvement interventions and technologies ranging from medicines labelling and technological alert systems, to teamwork checklists, and standardised communication tools. It has also led to calls for more proactive and systematic forms of organisational learning that help identify sources of error and target improvements, through forms of incident reporting and risk reduction.

Yet, we might question whether these ideas go far enough in understanding and explaining the latent factors that influence quality and safety, as well as the strength of their theoretical and methodological foundations. Much is made, for example, of 'the system', 'systemic factors' and 'systems thinking' within this orthodox paradigm, but the underlying conceptualisation of the 'system' is often less clear. In many examples, the application of systems thinking is limited to the 'micro-system' of clinical interactions, teamwork and environmental stressors, which without doubt have a bearing on the quality of care. But such an understanding of quality and safety frequently ignores the impact of wider social, cultural or organisational factors which impinge on healthcare practice. Although clinical and team behaviours might be enhanced by new procedures or reduced environmental stressors, it is important to recognise that these everyday practices are deeply social, being shaped by wider structures and cultural norms, such as professional jurisdictions, occupational hierarchies, gender differences, and status hierarchies. Mainstream approaches also frequently highlight the influence of cultural factors on healthcare quality and safety. There is little question that wider socio-cultural factors are important, and that the frequent calls for culture change are well-founded. However, from a sociological perspective, we might critique some of the simplistic understandings of culture on which much of the work in this area is founded and question the ease with which cultures can be changed. Much of the current interest in safety culture appears concerned with measuring espoused attitudes and behaviours through surveys or tools, without considering fully the underlying, often taken-for-granted meanings, beliefs and moral norms that also constitute cultures (Parker 2000). Similarly, the tendency for mainstream approaches to see systems of care in terms of linear cause-and-effect relationships and therefore amenable to re-engineering, is increasingly being challenged in the light of research which highlights the relational, cultural and technical complexity of healthcare systems (Allen 2014, Braithwaite 2006a, 2006b). Viewed from a sociological perspective, a host of salient mediating factors are neglected or poorly theorised within the orthodox view, such as the social structuring of activities and practice; the interactional character of care; social boundaries; organisational and professional cultures; the power dynamics of care delivery; and the regulatory, political and institutional contexts of care. The failure to sufficiently consider these wider social, cultural and institutional factors might explain why quality improvement interventions are challenging to implement or why successes made in one set-ting are difficult to replicate in another (Allen, in press).

Perhaps in light of these shortcomings, there is now a growing interest in better under-standing how 'context' influences the quality and safety of care, and the implementation of improvement interventions. The UK Health Foundation, for example, commissioned a col-lection of chapters on this topic (Bate *et al.* 2014). But as with the term 'culture' there is a risk that the concept of 'context' might also become an over-used and poorly understood catch-all term to explain all the intractable barriers to change. Social systems rarely follow linear models of causality, but involve multiple interacting (human and non-human) actors, oper-ating within specifically social circumstances and with relatively structured opportunities for agency, and where the patterns of interaction are simultaneously capable of reproducing and transforming the structured patterns of interaction and associated social and cultural systems. In short, while the words 'system', 'culture', and 'context' are common parlance in the field of quality and safety, deep understanding of this social, political and cultural com-plexity which sociology offers, is only recently coming to the fore. Thus notwithstanding the significant advances that have been made, mainstream perspectives have certain limitations and despite the apparent dominance of these ideas, there have been growing calls for alter-native perspectives (see Hollnagel *et al.* 2013, Wears *et al.* 2015) including that offered by sociology (Allen 2013a, in press, Rowley and Waring 2011).

Sociological contributions

Although sociological theory and research hitherto have made only marginal contributions to the mainstream paradigm, there is a rich and developed legacy on which current and future studies might draw. The publication of *Medical Nemesis* by Illich (1976) was a landmark soci-ological study of healthcare quality and safety. In this Marxist analysis of healthcare practice, Illich asserted that the medical profession had become a major threat to health and that the disabling impact of professional control over medicine had reached epidemic proportions. For Illich, medical errors had to be understood in the wider context of medical professional-ism, the institutionalisation of medical knowledge, and its impact on healthcare delivery. He drew attention to the alarming level and character of iatrogenic or 'medical-inflicted injuries' within contemporary healthcare systems stemming from the ineffective utility of medicine, mistakes in the delivery of care, unnecessary or over-treatment, and patient dependence on medical science:

> Among the murderous institutional torts, only modern malnutrition injures more people than iatrogenic disease in its various manifestations. (Illich 1976: 26)

Illich (1976: 30) recognised that medical errors can be checked or controlled through external mechanisms, such as litigation, but he argued that this is often complicated by the profession's ability to define the qualities of their work, especially by re-conceptualising medical faults as 'random human error' or 'system breakdown'. This work was significant, first, because it contributed to emerging sociological debates about professional power as articulated by Freidson (1970) and others, and second, because it spoke directly to the issues raised in the growing policy and clinical research community, but which paid little regard to the themes addressed by Illich, not least the critical questions he poses about the profession's ability to retain control of its practice through its power to frame the nature of the problem and thus its solution.

Yet to a considerable extent, mistakes are normal. To err really is human, and is especially likely in organisational settings where richly interactive relationships, intricate cultures and a bewildering range of systems, delivery mechanisms and agents co-produce unique episodes of care to a multiplicity of complex patients. Although not concerned exclusively with medicine or healthcare, an early sociological contribution illuminating this point lies with Hughes's (1951) analysis of mistakes at work. Hughes argued that all work tasks have the possibility of error, and as such, particular social relationships develop around tasks to accommodate and relocate these risks. With reference to specialist occupations, such as medicine, he suggests that client groups explicitly transfer the risk of mistake to an expert as a consequence of their own reduced expertise or skill. As well as highlighting the relational dimension of risk, his work also emphasised how definitions of mistake can be contested between specialist and client, but that such definitions are inherently framed by the asymmetries of knowledge and power. Hughes (1951: 323) acknowledged that in healthcare, categorising mistakes is often problematic because 'health is, after all, a relative matter'. These ideas suggest that classifications of patient safety, adverse incidents or medical errors are inevitably constructed within a social and cultural context; rather than fulfilling any objective or universal criteria. This might explain, for example, why reporting systems fail to capture certain experiences, why there are consistent discrepancies between professional groups, and how the definition of risk is often couched in terms of responsibility and blame (Swinglehurst *et al.* 2015, Waring 2005, 2009).

Hughes's ideas are developed further through Strauss *et al.*'s (1985) symbolic interactionist analysis of the social organisation of medical work. Grounded in a process view of organisations as negotiated orders and in a state of constant flux, their analysis examines the 'illness trajectory'[2] of patients to explore the complex and contingent nature of healthcare work. Through a number of case studies, the authors offer a detailed analysis of several inductively generated categories of work: sentimental work, machine work, safety work, body work, information work, comfort work, patients' work, and identity work. All are relevant to an understanding of quality and safety, but 'safety', 'sentimental' and 'articulation' work resonate most clearly with this agenda. What Strauss *et al.* reveal is that safety work has to be understood as integral to, and embedded in, everyday service delivery, where the responsibility for safety is distributed across the healthcare division of labour.

Like the scholarship of Hughes, the *Social Organization of Medical Work* is distinctive for its emphasis on healthcare work, rather than the workers. But as Illich signalled, any understanding of healthcare practice has to be grounded in an understanding of the institutional dominance of medicine. Freidson's (1970) analysis of medicine is a classic study in the sociology of health and illness, and locates questions about standards and quality within his understanding of professional autonomy and regulation. The medical profession's institutionalised control over its expert knowledge and its associated autonomy within the division of labour, has traditionally made it difficult for non-professionals to evaluate medical performance, thereby reinforcing claims to self-regulation:

The profession is the sole source of competence to recognise deviant performance and to regulate itself in general. Its autonomy is justified and tested by self-regulation. (Freidson 1970: 137)

This line of sociological analysis not only highlights how asymmetries of knowledge shape social interaction, but also how issues of quality and safety represent key sites of control and power within the social organisation of healthcare. This is supported by Arluke's (1977) discussion of symbolic control rituals in medical work, which shows how 'death rounds' constitute a social control ritual for normalising mistakes and maintaining the authority of medical professionalism. He describes, for example, how surgeons make sense of patient death in ways that de-emphasise its relationship with surgical performance.

One of the most important contributions to the sociological study of medical error is Bosk's *Forgive and Remember* (1979). This followed in the symbolic interactionist tradition to further develop the sociological analysis of professional socialisation (Becker *et al.* 1961, Davis and Olesen 1981, Dingwall 1977, Fox 1975, Lief and Fox 1963, Mumford 1970). His research explored how surgical trainees and their supervisors recognised, discussed and gave meaning to errors during the course of their surgical preparation, and how these formed the basis of social control rituals within professional socialisation. Bosk identified different social constructions of error including, 'technical' (procedural), 'judgement' (diagnostic) and 'normative' (conduct). In essence, he found 'judgement' and 'technical' mistakes served as valuable opportunities to assess the skills and abilities of the trainee, which were 'forgiven', but 'remembered' as part of the learning journey. 'Normative' mistakes, however, were used to assess the 'professional' character of trainees, such as their demeanour with patients or willingness to disclose mistakes, and were less easily excused. The philosophy behind medical training supported enhanced clinical exposure without excessive supervision, where mistakes become a 'regrettable but inevitable part of the baptism under fire that is house officer training' (Bosk 1986: 466). For Bosk, surgical training is a form of moral education centred on the standards of shared practice. In the recent re-publication of his work, Bosk (2003) acknowledges the growing patient safety movement and characterises efforts to improve safety as laudable. Reflecting on his work, he suggested change might be difficult. First, he reinforces the idea that safety and error are contested concepts and grounded in local knowledge, thereby eluding universal classification. Second, he argues that efforts to create a safety culture need to recognise that cultural elements do not exist in isolation, but rather operate amongst a wider milieu of meanings, values and customs. Third, he claims that the emphasis on 'near misses' is likely to be further complicated by contested nature of knowing but also a degree of hindsight bias, where some are regarded as trivial and others as potential disasters but where the gap between practices and outcome creates an uncertain space of knowing.

Although not explicitly related to the subject of medical errors, Fox (1975, 2000) also makes an interesting contribution to the sociology of quality and safety through questioning the supposed scientific conviction of medical knowledge. Specifically, she suggests that medical knowledge is characterised by 'gaps', inconsistencies and uncertainties around which cultural and occupational strategies have developed as a means of maintaining professional legitimacy, especially where these gaps are associated within unsafe practice. Fox described three types of uncertainty associated with, first, the difficulties of managing the vast knowledge and skills of modern medicine; second, the uncertainties that stem from inconsistencies in scientific knowledge; and third the problems associated with individual variations in skill and ability. Like Bosk (1979), she suggests professional socialisation facilitates the control of these uncertainties through, for example, the intellectualisation and definitional control of uncertainty. She also highlights a detached attitude towards uncertainty, which is regarded as a 'constant presence' but remains shrouded in silence. A similar line of thinking is found in Paget's (1988) phenomenological study of surgical error. This describes medical practice as characterised by a 'complex sorrow' in the context of almost inevitable patient harm.

A more recent sociological analysis of medical error is Rosenthal's (1995) study of 'problem doctors'. Building on the work of Bosk (1979) and Freidson (1970) she describes how the recognition and control of medical error is linked to wider dilemmas in medical knowledge and the demands of professionalism. In particular, she describes how doctors often find it difficult to define the boundaries between avoidable and unavoidable mistakes. Like Fox (1975) she suggests medical work is characterised by 'permanent uncertainty' which makes it possible for doctors to accept certain mistakes as 'necessary fallibility'. With this shared cultural sense of imperfection the medical profession exhibits a strong bond of collegiality, empathy, and togetherness that shapes how mistakes are controlled in everyday practice. Specifically, she describes a shared norm of 'non-criticism', which reinforces the idea of secrecy and conspiracy in medical work (Kennedy 2001). Nevertheless, it was also found that collegial acceptance has its limits and 'egregious errors' associated with gross misconduct or consistent misadventure, are not readily accepted.

Beyond healthcare, Green (1997) suggests there has been relatively little sociological writing on mistakes and accidents in everyday life; but the problems of organisational deviance have received considerable sociological attention and offer a powerful counterpoint to the mainstream approaches of safety science, e.g. high reliability theory (Perrow 1984, Turner 1978, Vaughan 1997). Perrow's (1984) work on *Normal Accidents* remains a major contribution to the field suggesting that accidents can be an inevitable or normal feature of organising. This is not because of the high-risk character of work or operator error, but because of the way tasks are organised so that 'discrete failures' cascade and escalate into more substantial disasters. This is elaborated along two lines. 'Interactive complexity' refers to the way commonplace problems, often located within organisational sub-systems, can interact and combine in unexpected ways to produce more profound accidents. Linked to this is an understanding of how organisational sub-systems are inter-dependent or 'tightly coupled' so that failures located within one process can spread across the wider system through a series of escalating knock-on effects. An organisation's structural arrangements can therefore transform risky or dangerous situations into disasters or normal accidents (Perrow 1984). This approach has been deployed in the healthcare context to explain, for example, the threats to safety in the operating theatre as a consequence of the tight couplings with other hospital departments (Waring *et al.* 1997).

This organisational perspective is developed further in Vaughan's (1999) work on the Challenger Space Shuttle disaster. Building on Merton's (1970) notion of bureaucratic dysfunction, she elaborates a sociology of organisational 'dark sides' that relates individual performance and cognition, to the role of teams, system processes, organisational structures and the wider environment or structures of society. This area of sociological work is significant because it addresses explicitly the meso and macro dimensions of safety, rather than the more micro world of group psychology, technology and practice. West (2000) develops this approach to elaborate four 'dark sides' of healthcare organisation. This includes, first, the 'division of labour' and rigid demarcations between occupational roles, expertise and responsibility that run counter to the desired objectives of integrated working. Second, healthcare services have a 'homophilic' character, which encourages occupational groups to interact with those most like themselves, thereby reducing integration and inhibiting communication. Third, problems in the delivery of healthcare are not adequately addressed because of the 'diffusion of responsibility' where potential problems are seen as somebody else's responsibility. Fourth, 'goal displacement' where multiple and competing priorities relocate the focus of action towards activities that may be more prone to mistake or less concerned with quality.

Sociologists have also offered critical insights into more recent developments in the healthcare quality and safety movement, and have pressed the point that these problems cannot be resolved through mere technological innovation, linear interventions or increased vigilance.

For example, Wiener (2000) examined efforts in the US to increase hospital care quality through enhanced standardisation of work. Drawing on extensive observational work in two hospitals she concludes that many aspects of care defy standardisation, and as such, this quest will always remain elusive. McDonald and colleagues (2006) similarly examined attitudes of clinicians and managers in the English National Health Service about standardisation, concluding that these groups not only had vastly different identities, histories and characteristics but they proceeded on the basis of entirely different world-views. Specifically, the medical perspective opposed standardisation, advocated the legitimacy of clinical judgement, and tolerated uncertainty and risk. The managerial discourse, on the other hand, sought standardisation, adherence to guidelines, and underpinned their activities with a claim – perhaps a hope – that structured, linear, rational solutions could be successfully applied to complex socio-professional environments. Fundamentally, doctors believed quality and safety was an art and managers thought it was a science. They conclude that the dominant paradigm simply cannot deliver on its promises. In *The Gold Standard* Timmermans and Berg (2003) address similar concerns, but reach quite different conclusions. Rather than rejecting all efforts of standardisation they argue: 'just what accountability should look like, whose burden it is to carry it and whose to demand it, what information should satisfy this request, and so forth are the very conflicts that are *settled* in and through the creation of standards […] the issue is not *whether* procedural standardisation is good or possible, but *how* it should be put to work' (Timmermans and Berg 2003: 201–2, original emphasis). There is a growing body of sociological work which has taken up this challenge (Allen 2004, 2013, Gabbay and Le May 2004, Moreira 2005, Pinder *et al.* 2005, Timmermans and Berg 1997).

Another sociological challenge to the orthodox paradigm centres on a critique of the 'deficit model' and its preoccupation with error. Although research might suggest 10 per cent of hospital care is 'unsafe', there has been little consideration of the practices that make up to 90 per cent of the 'safe' care including the 'rescue work' of professionals (Waring *et al.* 2007). Through a process of 'exnovation', Mesman's (2011) programme of research in neonatal intensive care units uncovers the informal and unarticulated work involved in preserving clinical safety. This draws attention to the everyday skills through which quality and safety is maintained and the practical wisdom that contributes to organisational resilience. While Mesman's focus is on clinical skills in a specialist and relatively 'high tech' environment, recent work by Allen (2014) has drawn attention to the everyday 'organising work' of hospital nurses and its contribution to quality and patient safety. She argues that nurses are the obligatory passage points in healthcare systems who, through their everyday organising work, funnel, refract and shape all the activity that contributes to patient care, through a process she terms, 'translational mobilisation'. This work is poorly understood and relatively invisible to the formal organisation. Others have also highlighted the contribution of backstage work in supporting healthcare quality and safety (Iedema *et al.* 2006).

As well as a preoccupation with errors and the application of technical solutions, as we have seen, the orthodox paradigm has also emphasised the importance of 'culture management'. For example, policies repeatedly talk of replacing a 'blame culture' with a 'safety culture' that is attentive to risk, open and transparent, and responsive to improvement systems (Donaldson 2000). Jensen (2008) has scrutinised such efforts and argued that, to the sociologically minded, trying to change 'culture' is improbable at best; a point also highlighted by Bosk (2003). With multiple stakeholders, complex hierarchies and heterarchies, conflicting world views and politically-charged environments all affecting and, indeed, comprising the embedded cultures of healthcare, simplistic calls for culture change are infeasible. From this perspective, conceptualising patient safety and quality of care as a problem of systems redesign that is amenable to a 'cause-and-effect' logic, is not just a bad idea, it is irrational:

> [A] realistic analysis of healthcare must simultaneously deal with its intertwined social and professional, cultural and political, scientific and technical facets. Adverse events, for example, are surely not just (or primarily) due to human error at the ward level but are rather a systemic – or networked – consequence of the ways in which health work is related to cultures or management, governance, business and science. (Jensen 2008: 322)

Discussion

The dominant approach to healthcare quality and safety has made important contributions to how policy, research and practice understand and seek to improve the organisation and delivery of patient care. In particular, it has shifted attention away from individual error to bring to light the common latent factors that many healthcare professionals and patients face. It has also made important breakthroughs through the development and implementation of safety-enhancing or quality improvement interventions and technologies. Yet these ideas only go so far in accounting for the wider social, cultural and institutional factors that influence the quality and safety of care, about which sociological insights have the potential to complement and extend the mainstream perspectives. Take for example, the assumption that a common set of ideas, techniques and tools for improvement can be translated from other high-risk industries and adopted, almost regardless of context, to enhance care quality. Sociology dispels this illusion of control. Instead it has shown the need to unravel the multiple dimensions of quality and safety (Braithwaite and Coiera 2010, Dixon-Woods 2010), and apprehend its context-bound nature (Plumb 2013) in which quality and safety are understood as emergent products of distributed stakeholder relationships and assemblages of people, materials and ideas (Latour 2005, Mol 2002). In this view safety and quality are multiple and contested 'processes-in-the-making' rather than static states or concrete edifices amenable to external manipulation.

Reflecting on these currents of sociological thought, Waring (2013) outlines three linked dilemmas in understanding healthcare safety and quality, where the 'nested' relationship between these might be conceived as a type of Russian doll. The first dilemma relates to the epistemology of quality and safety, specifically the tendency of dominant approaches towards abstraction and concretisation. This can be seen in the ways policy and research present risks as explicit, real and tangible 'events' that can be understood and measured through objective enquiry and systematic analysis, including the use of taxonomies and classification tools. This realist perspective stands in contrast to a constructionist sociological viewpoint, which sees meanings of, and responses to, clinical risks as the product of shared relationships, attitudes and beliefs, conflicting discourses and social conventions. Whereas the former supposes that knowledge about safety can be objectively communicated, for example through incident reporting, the latter suggests that knowledge is inherently situated in practices, framed by wider cultural frames, and linked to institutionalised lines of power (Waring 2009).

The second dilemma centres on culture, and the way culture is conceived and operationalised as a source of (un)safety. The dominant paradigm often takes the view that 'culture' is something that a healthcare organisation 'has'; which is amenable to both abstract measurement and change. Alternatively, sociologists recognise culture as something that an organisation 'is'; as a property of underlying social structures and emerging through social

interactions that are intrinsically infused with differences, shifting conflicts and variable attitudes, values and predispositions, such that within complex organisations with their var-
iegated workshops (Strauss *et al.* 1985) and social groups it makes more sense to talk of
organisational culture*s* (Braithwaite *et al.* 2010, Hughes and Allen 1993).

The third dilemma centres on power and politics. The orthodox approach is that healthcare settings can be rendered politically benign or even depoliticised by appropriate effort
such as team building activities. Many of the strategies aimed at implementing quality
improvement interventions focus on the fidelity of the intervention, the appropriateness of
the intervention to the setting, and wider contextual factors (e.g. Damschroder *et al.* 2009,
Greenhalgh *et al.* 2004). However, this can neglect the inherent political and ideological
dynamics of healthcare organisations, especially where established ways of working reflect
the institutionalised power of certain actors or professions (see Nugus *et al.* 2010). Improvement interventions inevitably involve changing the established ways of working, customary
practices, and shared identities that are constituted by, and reinforcing of, prevailing forms of
power and authority. This explains why so often quality improvements are resisted by vested
interests (Waring and Currie 2009) and the need for enhanced political acuity in improvement
processes to enable the recognition and mediation of institutional power relationships.

In each of these dilemmas, the difference between the dominant paradigm and the sociological perspective signals a potential future direction of travel for sociological contributions
to the wicked problem (Churchman 1967) of healthcare safety and quality. Yet a more thor-
oughgoing engagement with these concerns also raises questions about the nature of the discipline's engagement with this policy priority and the uses to which sociological work is put.
For some, understanding quality and safety in these terms opens up possibilities for positive
engagement between sociology and the quality movement. For example, in their epilogue
to *The Gold Standard,* Timmermans and Berg (2003) see a close alignment between more
sociological insights and the orthodox view developed within *To Err is Human* (Institute of
Medicine 1999) and argue for sociologists to be part of, rather than above, the networks they
study. Others have also challenged the social sciences community to move beyond critiques
of patient safety and collaborate more actively with clinicians and patient safety researchers
(Vincent 2009). As outlined above, there is an emerging cadre of researchers who are developing new approaches to engaging with the quality improvement agenda. Notable examples
include work on video-reflexivity (Iedema *et al.* 2013), emerging models of acting with quality
improvers in healthcare (Zuiderent-Jerak *et al.* 2009) and ideas drawn from resilient engineering (Hollnagel *et al.* 2013, Waring 2013, Wears *et al.* 2015). There is also a growing realisation
of the potential contribution of social science concepts and perspectives in developing the
theoretical basis for improvement efforts (Davidoff *et al.* 2014, Dixon-Woods *et al.* 2011).
As Jensen (2008) observes, however, one of the consequences of *To Err is Human* has been
to focus attention on health professional practice as a core concern, to the neglect of wider
aspects of the healthcare system: social, bureaucratic, economic and political. Whilst there is
much to commend the alignment of sociologists with this agenda, the work of social science
needs to be more than that of uncovering those factors which help or hinder the implementation of quality and safety policy. Indeed, one of the core strengths of sociology of quality
and safety is its potential to stand outside dominant framings and offer an alternative lens.

In this chapter we have traced the evolution of the healthcare quality and safety movement across four waves of development. We have argued that it is only in the last three decades
that the topic has gained policy momentum across international arena and this has driven
research and practice in this field. Despite healthcare quality and safety being topics of central sociological concern, for the best part of its development, scholarship has developed
largely outside of mainstream quality and safety research and practice. There are signs that

this is changing and it is possible to identify the dilemmas in the current orthodoxy to which the accumulating body of sociological work might contribute. While there is both an opportunity for and a willingness to embrace more integrated working in this field, this is not without its challenges, raising a dilemma familiar to medical sociologists as to whether we should be advancing a sociology *of* quality and safety or developing a sociology for quality and safety.

Acknowledgements

Jane Sandall was supported by the National Institute for Health Research (NIHR) Collaboration for Leadership in Applied Health Research and Care South London at King's College Hospital NHS Foundation Trust. Justin Waring was supported by the National Institute for Health Research (NIHR) Collaboration for Leadership in Applied Health Research and Care East Midlands. The views expressed are those of the author(s) and not necessarily those of the NHS, the NIHR or the Department of Health.

Notes

1   The Swiss Cheese Model of accident causation likens human systems to multiple slices of Swiss cheese in that risks and threats are mitigated by the layering effects of different kinds of defences, to prevent a single point of weakness. The model was originally developed by Dante Orlandella and James T Reason.
2   The term refers 'not only to the physiological unfolding of a patient's disease but to the total organization of work done over that course, plus the impact on those involved with that work and its organization' (Strauss *et al.* 1985: 8).

References

Allen, D. (2009) From boundary concept to boundary object: the politics and practices of care pathway development, *Social Science and Medicine*, 69, 3, 354–61.
Allen, D. (2013a) Situated context for quality improvement purposes: artefacts, affordances and socio-technical infrastructure, *Health*, 15, 5, 460–77.
Allen, D. (2013b) The sociology of carework, Sociology of Health Illness Virtual Special Issue: The Francis Series. Available at http://onlinelibrary.wiley.com/journal/10.1111/(ISSN)1467-9566/ homepage/ the_sociology_of_care.htm. Date last accessed 1 December 2015.
Allen, D. (2014) *The Invisible Work of Nurses: Hospitals, Organisation and Healthcare.* London and New York: Routledge.
Arluke, A. (1977) 'Social control rituals in medicine: the case of death rounds'. In Dingwall, R., Heath, C., Reid, M. and Stacey, M. (eds) *Health Care and Health Knowledge.* London: Croom Helm.
Baker, G.R., Norton, P.G., Flintoft, V., Blais, R., *et al.* (2004) The Canadian adverse events study: the incidence of adverse events among hospital patients in Canada, *CMAJ*, 170, 11, 1678–86.
Bate, P., Robert, G., Fulop, N., Ovretveit, J., *et al.* (2014) *Perspectives on Context: A Selection of Essays Considering the Role of Context in Successful Quality Improvement.* London: The Health Foundation.
Becker, A.S., Geer, B., Hughes, E.C. and Strauss, A.L. (1961) *Boys in White: Student Culture in Medical School.* Chicago, IL: University of Chicago Press.
Bosk, C. (1979) *Forgive and Remember: Managing Error: The Culture of Safety on the Shop Floor.* Princeton, NJ: Institute for Advanced Study.

Bosk, C. (1986) Professional responsibility and medical error. In Aiken, L. and Mechanic, D. (eds) *Applications in Social Science to Clinical Medicine and Health Policy.* Brunswick, NJ: Rutgers University Press.

Bosk, C. (2003) *Forgive and Remember: Managing Medical Failure*, 2nd edn. London: University of Chicago Press.

Braithwaite, J. (2006a) Analysing structural and cultural change in acute settings using a Giddens-Weick paradigmatic approach, *Health Care Analysis*, 14, 2, 91–102.

Braithwaite, J. (2006b) An empirical assessment of social structural and cultural change in clinical directorates, *Health Care Analysis*, 14, 4, 185–93.

Braithwaite, J. and Coiera, E. (2010) Beyond patient safety flatland, *Journal of the Royal Society of Medicine*, 103, 6, 219–25.

Braithwaite, J., Hyde, P. and Pope, C. (eds) (2010) *Culture and Climate in Health Care Organisations.* London: Palgrave Macmillan.

Braithwaite, J., Clay-Williams, R., Nugus, P. and Plumb, J. (2013) Health care as a complex adaptive system. In Hollnagel, E., Braithwaite, J. and Wears, R. (eds) *Resilient Health Care.* Farnham: Ashgate.

Brennan, T. and Leape, L. (1991) Incidence of adverse events and negligence in hospitalized patients, *New England Journal of Medicine*, 324, 6, 370–6.

Bulger, R.J. (ed) (1973) *Hippocrates Revisited: A Search for Meaning.* New York: Medcom Press.

Cassirere, C. and Anderson, D. (2004) Future of patient safety: reflections on history, the data and what it will take to succeed. In Youngberb, B.J. and Hatlie, M.J. (eds) *Patient Safety Handbook.* Sudbury, MA: Jones and Barlett Publishers.

Churchman, C.W. (1967) Wicked Problems, *Management Science*, 14, 4, 141–2.

Codman, E.A. (1917) *A Study in Hospital Efficiency: as Demonstrated by the Case Report of the First Five Years of a Private Hospital.* Oak Brook, IL: Joint Commission Resources.

Cohen, S. (2002) *Folk Devils and Moral Panics: The Creation of the Mods and Rockers.* London: Psychology Press.

Damschroder, L.J., Aron, D.C., Keith, R.E., Kirsh, S.R., *et al.* (2009) Fostering implementation of health services research findings into practice: a consolidated framework for advancing implementation science, *Implementation Science*, 4, 1, 50.

Davidoff, F., Dixon-Woods, M., Leviton, L. and Michie, S. (2014) Demystifying theory and its use in improvement, *BMJ Quality and Safety*, 24, 3, 228–38.

Davis, F. and Olesen, V. (1981) Initiation into a woman's profession: identity problems in the status transition of coed to student nurse, *Sociometry*, 22, 1, 29–33.

Davis, P., Lay-Yee, R., Briant, R., Schug, S., *et al.* (2002) *Adverse Events in New Zealand Public Hospitals: Principle Findings from a National Survey.* Wellington, New Zealand: Ministry of Health.

Dingwall, R. (1977) *The Social Organisation of Health Visitor Training.* London: Croom Helm.

Dixon-Woods, M. (2010) Why is patient safety so hard?, *A selective review of ethnographic studies, Journal of Health Services Research and Policy*, 15, 1, 1–16.

Dixon-Woods, M., Bosk, C.L., Aveling, E.L., Goeschel, C.A., *et al.* (2011) Explaining Michigan: developing an ex post theory of a quality improvement program, *The Milbank Quarterly*, 89, 2, 167–205.

Donabedian, A. (2003) *An Introduction to Quality Assurance in Healthcare.* New York: Oxford University Press.

Donaldson, L. (2000) *An Organization with a Memory.* London: The Stationary Office.

Ehrich, K. (2006) Telling cultures: 'cultural' issues for staff reporting concerns about colleagues in the UK National Health Service, *Sociology of Health & Illness*, 28, 7, 903–26.

Fox, R.C. (1975) Training for uncertainty. In Cox, C. and Mead, A. (eds) *A Sociology of Medical Practice.* London: Collier-MacMillan.

Fox, R. (2000) Medical uncertainty revisited. In Albrecht, G., Fitzgerald, R. and Scrimshaw, S. (eds) *Handbook of Social Studies in Health and Medicine.* London: Sage.

Freidson, E. (1970) *Professional Dominance.* New York: Atherton Press.

Freidson, E. (1975) *Doctoring Together: A Study of Professional Social Control.* New York: Elsevier.

Francis, R. (Chair) (2013) *The Mid Staffordshire NHS Foundation Trust Public Inquiry; vol 1: Analysis of Evidence and Lessons Learned (part 1).* London: TSO.

Gabbay, J. and Le May, A. (2004) Evidence based guidelines or collectively constructed "mindlines?" Ethnographic study of knowledge management in primary care, *British Medical Journal*, 329, 7473, 1013–6.

Green, J. (1997) *Risk and Misfortune: The Social Construction of Accidents*. London: UCL Press.

Greenhalgh, T., Robert, G., Macfarlane, F., Bate, P., *et al.* (2004) Diffusion of innovations in service organizations: systematic review and recommendations, *Milbank Quarterly*, 82, 4, 581–629.

Hindle, D., Braithwaite, J., Iedema, R. and Travaglia, J. (2006) *Patient Safety: A Comparative Analysis of Eight Inquiries in Six Countries*. Sydney: University of New South Wales.

Hollnagel, E., Braithwaite, J. and Wears, R.L. (eds) (2013) *Resilient Health Care*. Farnham: Ashgate.

Hughes, D. (2013) Sociological Perspectives on Regulation and Governance, The Francis Reports Virtual Special Issue Series: Care Standards, Regulation and Accountability. Available at http://onlinelibrary.wiley.com/journal/10.1111/(ISSN)1467-9566/homepage/sociological_perspectives_on_regulation_and_governance.htm. Date last accessed 1 December 2015.

Hughes, D. and Allen, D. (1993) Inside the Black Box: Obstacles to Change in the Modern Hospital Kings Fund and Milbank Memorial Fund, Joint Health Policy Review. Kings-Fund: London.

Hughes, D. and Light, D. (eds) (2002) *Rationing: Constructed Realities and Professional Practices*. Oxford: Wiley-Blackwell.

Hughes, E.C. (1951) 'Mistakes at work', reprinted in Hughes, E.C. (1971) *The Sociological Eye*. Chicago, IL: Aldine Atherton.

Iedema, R., Long, D., Carroll, K., Stenglin, M., *et al.* (2006) Corridor work: how luminal spaces becomes a resource for handling complexities of multidisciplinary healthcare, Pacific Researchers in Organizational Studies 11th Colloquium, 238-47. Available at http://search.informit.com.au/documentSummary;dn=305691933675194;res=IELBUS (accessed 27 July 2015).

Iedema, R., Mesman, J. and Carroll, J. (eds) (2013) *Visualising Health Care Practice Improvement: Innovation From Within*. London: Radcliffe Health.

Illich, I. (1976) *Medical Nemesis: The Exploration of Health*. New York: Pantheon Books.

Institute of Medicine (1999) *To Err is Human*. Washington, DC: National Academy of Sciences.

Institute of Medicine (2001) *Crossing the Quality Chasm: A New Health System for the 21st Century*. Washington, DC: National Academy of Sciences.

Jensen, C.B. (2008) Sociology, systems and (patient) safety; knowledge translations in healthcare policy, *Sociology of Health & Illness*, 30, 12, 309–24.

Jones, A. and Kelly, D. (2014) Whistle-blowing and workplace culture in older peoples' care: qualitative insights from the healthcare and social care workforce, *Sociology of Health & Illness*, 36, 7, 986–1002.

Kennedy, I. (Chair) (2001) *Learning from Bristol*. London: TSO.

Larson, M.S. (2013) *The Rise of Professionalism*. London: Transaction Books.

Latour, B. (2005) *Reassembling the Social*. Oxford: Oxford University Press.

Le Fanu, J. (2011) *The Rise and Fall of Modern Medicine*. London: Little Brown Book Group.

Leape, L. and Brennan, T. (1991) The nature of adverse events in hospitalized patients, *New England Journal of Medicine*, 324, 6, 377–84.

Lief, H.I. and Fox, R.C. (1963) Training for "detached concern" in medical students. In Lief, H., Lief, V.F. and Lief, N.R. (eds) *The Psychological Basis of Medical Practice*. New York: Harper and Row.

Lindsay, P., Sandall, J. and Humphrey, C. (2012) The social dimensions of safety incident reporting in maternity care: the influence of working relationships and group processes, *Social Science & Medicine*, 75, 10, 1793–9.

Marshall, M., Pronovost, P. and Dixon-Woods, M. (2013) View point: promotion of improvement as a science, *Lancet*, 381, 9864, 419–21.

McDonald, R., Waring, J. and Harrison, S. (2006) Rules, safety and narrativisation of identity: a hospital operating theatre case study, *Sociology of Health & Illness*, 28, 2, 178–202.

Merton, R. (1970) Bureaucratic structure and personality. In Etzioni, A. (ed) *Sociological Reader on Complex Organizations*. London: HRW.

Mesman, J. (2011) *Uncertainty in Medical Innovation: Experienced Pioneers in Neonatal Care*. Basingstoke: Palgrave Macmillan.

Mol, A. (2002) *The Body Multiple: Ontology in Medical Practice*. Durham, NC: Duke University Press.

Moreira, T. (2005) Diversity in clinical guidelines: the role of repertoires of evaluation, *Social Science & Medicine*, 60, 9, 1975–85.

Mumford, E. (1970) *Interns: From Students to Physicians.* Cambridge, MA: Harvard University Press.

Nugus, P., Greenfield, D., Travaglia, J., Westbrook, J., *et al.* (2010) How and where clinicians exercise power: interprofessional relations in health care, *Social Science & Medicine*, 71, 5, 898–909.

Paget, M. (1988) *The Unity of Mistakes.* Philadelphia, PA: Temple University Press.

Parker, M. (2000) *Organisational Culture and Identity.* London: Sage.

Perrow, C. (1984) *Normal Accidents: Living with High-risk Technologies.* Princeton, NJ: Princeton University Press.

Pinder, R., Petchey, R., Shaw, S. and Carter, Y. (2005) What's in a care pathway? Towards a cultural cartography of the new NHS, *Sociology of Health & Illness*, 27, 6, 759–79.

Plumb, J. (2013) Taming uncertainty, performance, personalization and practices of patient safety in an Australian mental health service. Unpublished PhD dissertation. Sydney: University of New South Wales.

Porter, R. (1997) *The Greatest Benefit to Mankind: A Medical History of Humanity from Antiquity to the Present.* London: HarperCollins.

Power, M. (1997) *The Audit Society: Rituals of Verification.* Oxford: Oxford University Press.

Raju, T.N. (1999) Ignaz Semmelweis and the etiology of fetal and neonatal sepsis, *Journal of Perinatology*, 19, 4, 307–10.

Reason, J. (2000) Human error: models and management, *British Medical Journal*, 320, 7237, 768–70.

Rosenthal, M. (1995) *The Incompetent Doctor.* Buckingham: Open Press University.

Sharpe, V.A. and Faden, A.I. (1998) *Medical Harm: Historical, Conceptual and Ethical Dimensions of Iatrogenic Illness.* Cambridge: Cambridge University Press.

Small, S.D. and Barach, P. (2002) Patient safety and health policy: a history and a review, *Haematology and Oncology Clinics of North America*, 16, 6, 1463–82.

Smith, J. (Chair) (2005) *The Shipman Inquiry: Sixth Report – the Final Report.* London: TSO.

Spector, M. and Kituse, J. (2009) *Constructing Social Problems.* London: Transaction Publishers.

Stanley, N. and Manthorpe, J. (2004) *The Age of Inquiry: Learning and Blaming in Health and Social Care.* London: Routledge.

Stetson, H.G. and Moran, J.E. (1934) Malpractice suits, their cause and prevention, *New England Journal of Medicine*, 210, 26, 1381–5.

Strauss, A.L., Fagerhaugh, S., Suczek, B. and Wiener, C. (1985) *Social Organization of Medical Work.* Chicago, IL: University of Chicago Press.

Swinglehurst, D., Emmerich, N., Maybin, J., Park, S., *et al.* (2015) The many meanings of 'quality' in healthcare: interdisciplinary perspectives, *BMC Health Services Research*, 15, 240.

Timmermans, S. and Berg, M. (1997) Standardization in action: achieving local universality through medical protocols, *Social Studies of Science*, 27, 2, 273–305.

Timmermans, S. and Berg, M. (2003) *The Gold Standard: The Challenge of Evidence-based Medicine and Standardization in Health Care.* Philadelphia, PA: Temple University Press.

Travaglia, J.F. (2009) *Locating vulnerability in the field of patient safety: Unpublished PhD dissertation.* Sydney: University of New South Wales.

Turner, B.A. (1978) *Man Made Disasters.* London: Wykeham Science Press.

Vaughan, D. (1997) *The Challenger Launch Decision: Risky Technology, Culture and Deviance at NASA.* Chicago, IL: University of Chicago Press.

Vaughan, D. (1999) The dark side of organizations: Mistake, misconduct, and disaster, *Annual Review of Sociology*, 25, 271–305.

Vincent, C. (2006) *Patient Safety.* Edinburgh: Elsevier.

Vincent, C. (2009) Social scientists and patient safety: Critics or contributors? *Social Science & Medicine*, 69, 12, 1777–9.

Vincent, C., Neale, G. and Woloshynowych, M. (2001) Adverse events in British hospitals: preliminary retrospective record review, *British Medical Journal*, 322, 7285, 517–9.

Walshe, K. (2003) *Regulating Health Care: Prescriptions for Improvement.* Maidenhead: Open University Press.

Waring, J. (2005) Beyond blame: cultural barriers to medical incident reporting, *Social Science and Medicine*, 60, 9, 1927–35.

Waring, J. (2007) Adaptive regulation or governmentality: patient safety and the changing regulation of medicine, *Sociology of Health & Illness*, 29, 2, 163–79.

Waring, J. (2009) Constructing and re-constructing narratives of patient safety, *Social Science & Medicine*, 69, 12, 1722–31.

Waring, J. (2013) What safety-II might learn from the socio-cultural critique of safety-I. In Hollnagel, E., Braithwaite, J. and Wears, R. (eds) *Resilient Health Care*. Farnham: Ashgate.

Waring, J. and Currie, G. (2009) Managing expert knowledge: organizational challenges and managerial futures for the UK medical profession, *Organization Studies*, 30, 7, 755–78.

Waring, J. and Rowley, E. (2011) Introduction: a socio-cultural perspective on patient safety. In Rowley, E. and Waring, J. (eds) *A Socio-cultural Perspective on Patient Safety*. Farnham: Ashgate.

Waring, J., Harrison, S. and McDonald, R. (1997) Culture of safety or coping?, Ritualistic behaviours in the operating department, *Journal of Health Services Research and Policy*, 12, 1, 3–9.

Wears, R.L., Hollnagel, E. and Braithwaite, J. (2015) *Resilient Health Care, Volume 2: The Resilience of Everyday Clinical Work*. Farnham: Ashgate.

Wennberg, J.E. (1984) Dealing with medical practice variations: a proposal for action, *Health Affairs*, 3, 2, 6–32.

West, E. (2000) Organisational sources of safety and danger: sociological contributions to the study adverse events, *Quality and Safety in Healthcare*, 9, 2, 120–6.

Wiener, C. (2000) *The Elusive Quest: Accountability in Hospitals*. New York: Aldine de Gruyter.

Wilson, R.M., Runciman, W.B., Gibberd, R.W., Harrison, B.T., *et al.* (1995) The quality in Australian health care study, *Medical Journal of Australia*, 163, 9, 458–71.

Zuiderent-Jerak, T., Strating, M., Niebor, A. and Bar, R. (2009) Sociological reconfigurations of patient safety; ontologies of improvement and 'acting with' quality collaboratives in healthcare, *Social Science & Medicine*, 69, 12, 1731–21.

3

What is the role of individual accountability in patient safety? A multi-site ethnographic study

Emma-Louise Aveling, Michael Parker and Mary Dixon-Woods

Introduction

Though more than 15 years have passed since the birth of the modern patient safety movement (Kohn *et al.* 2000), one of its most important debates endures: how to distribute responsibility between organisational systems and individual professionals. The early phase of the movement was dominated by the view that error was not the result of individual failing, but instead was an inescapable feature of poorly designed systems. Accordingly, it was argued individuals should not be blamed for safety lapses: the proper response was said to involve the re-engineering of systems to avert or mitigate error (Leape *et al.* 2000). More recently, this so-called 'systems' approach has been argued to result in an unwarranted, misguided and risky attribution of all responsibility for safety to systems (Wachter and Pronovost 2009). A 'just culture' rather than a no-blame approach is now increasingly advocated, amid calls for individuals and systems both to be accountable and for those accountabilities to be balanced (Wachter 2013).

The question of how to allocate responsibility between systems and individuals has important instrumental value: it is of critical practical relevance because getting it wrong may undermine safety. Disciplining individuals who make errors in contexts of inadequately designed or poorly functioning systems may occlude deep organisational or institutional pathologies. Searching for systems defects when an individual is at fault may be an equally fruitless effort. Yet current prescriptions for the making of judgements to support a just culture draw upon only a limited evidence-base (empirical and theoretical) and tend to be prescriptive and mechanistic. One widely-cited 'algorithm' for determining the responsibility of individuals, for example, distinguishes between three types of error (human error, reckless behaviour, and at-risk behaviour) and matches them to a proposed response (consoling, punishment, and coaching, respectively) (Marx 2001). Another decision-tool uses a 'culpability tree' (Meadows *et al.* 2005) to guide users through a series of questions about the individual's actions, motives and behaviour at the time of the incident. These formulas have been criticised for their essentialist assumption that some acts or behaviours are inherently culpable and for their supposition that the making of distinctions between the acceptable and the unacceptable can be rendered tractable to simple rules (Dekker 2012). They may be therefore ill-suited even to the instrumental task of improving the effectiveness of patient safety efforts.

The problems with this calculus-like approach go far deeper, however. First, in their preoccupation with instrumental value, they tend to diminish the intrinsic value of an explicit

The Sociology of Healthcare Safety and Quality, First Edition. Edited by Davina Allen, Jeffrey Braithwaite, Jane Sandall and Justin Waring. Chapters © 2016 The Authors. Book Compilation © 2016 Foundation for the Sociology of Health & Illness/Blackwell Publishing Ltd.

emphasis on the moral agency of individuals. The idea that there is an inherent good in asking people to be good goes back to antiquity, but it is one that has special valence for the healthcare professions. The term 'profession' has been linked to virtues – such as benevolence, compassion, mercy and competence – since the earliest usage of the term (Pellegrino 2002). Recent years have seen renewed sociological attention – from previously sceptical quarters – to the social function and value of a morally-founded conceptualisation of the professions, accompanied by warnings of the dangers of its diminishment (Brint 2006, Freidson 2001).

Second, calculus-like approaches promote an asocial, atomistic and static account, one that neglects long-standing sociological insights about the scope, nature and possibilities of the individual agency of situated actors in institutionalised settings. In the field of organisation studies, such insights are increasingly gathered under the rubric of 'practice theory', which promotes an understanding of organisational phenomena as 'dynamic and accomplished in ongoing, everyday actions … we understand the mutually constitutive ways in which agency is shaped by but also produces, reinforces and changes its structural conditions' (Feldman and Orlikowski 2011: 1250). In offering this account of the emergent constitution of the social world through routine practices in organisations, practice theory explicitly invokes a rich sociological heritage, including (though not only) Giddens's (1984: 26) conceptualisation of structure and agency as a duality, mutually reinforcing and in constant dynamic interaction, such that the 'moment of production of action is also one of reproduction'. On this view, structure creates and shapes the possibilities for agency, at the same time as agency creates and shapes structure.

Positioning individuals as knowledgeable agents who reflexively monitor the flow of interactions with one another, Giddens (1984: 30) introduces a notion of accountability that emphasises the answerability of actors in terms of norms: 'To be "accountable" for one's activities is both to explicate the reasons for them and to supply the normative grounds whereby they may be "justified"'. He also notes that such norms cannot readily be programmed externally (for example through codes of conduct); instead normative expectations are socially contingent and must be sustained through the effective mobilisation of sanctions during actual encounters. Accordingly, for actors in specific social environments, what is deemed right and proper conduct is likely to be far more influenced by norms and values as they are produced and reproduced within those environments than they are by external standards and codifications. For those seeking to examine patient safety, a critical set of tasks therefore focuses on characterising how the work of healthcare gets done, how the norms, routines and institutionalised practices of organisational settings allocate responsibility and facilitate distinctions between blameless and blameworthy actions, and how, by whom and to whom the available sanctions are applied.

These are the tasks that *Forgive and Remember,* Bosk's (2003) classic ethnography assumes. Though he does not use the term 'practice theory' explicitly (the term was developed subsequent to his work), Bosk's study of surgeons-in-training vividly demonstrates the salience of that literature. He identifies how norms of responsibility are articulated and enforced through repeated and collectivised patterns of noticing, recognising, explaining, and disciplining actions and events. He shows how individuals are made accountable for what they do through processes of social control that, crucially, do not shrink from the imputation of blame: some errors may be deemed 'forgivable' but others taken as evidence of moral failing. Among the less forgivable errors are those that fail to honour the commitments that the profession requires; these errors are both sanctionable and sanctioned.

In calling out the importance of blame and punishment, *Forgive and Remember* disrupts the narrative of default blamelessness associated with the systems approach to patient safety, but it continues a sociological tradition dating back to Durkheim about the value of sanctioning as a collective responsibility that helps to make visible and reinforce the norms of a community (including a professional community) and to increase solidarity with that community. Bosk also makes another crucial, and under-recognised, observation. He shows that while near-universal consensus may exist on the culpability of some behaviours and actions, another class of apparent violations – termed 'quasi-normative' errors – involves failure to comply with senior physicians' personal preferences. This apparently more capricious category makes the broader point that situated agents may not themselves agree on what constitutes good practice. If calculus-like approaches are limited by their simplistic and flawed assumptions, and leaving it up to agents in their own environments susceptible to arbitrariness, then alternative ways of reasoning about how to draw boundaries around the accountabilities of individuals are needed. We suggest that concepts and reasoning from the ethics and political science literatures have much to offer in this regard.

A first and basic question concerns the extent to which individuals qualify as having responsibility for which they are answerable (and are thus accountable). We propose that to be held accountable, a moral agent must know of the standards she is expected to meet, be charged with responsibility for meeting those standards, and have sufficient autonomy and capacity in her choice of actions, and access to resources, to be able to comply: 'ought implies can' (Kant 1973). Assessments of accountability thus need to be attentive to the constraints on choices and actions, and to the nature of those constraints.

A second question concerns how to identify individual contributions to patient safety given that the potential contributors may be multiple and widely diffused, for example across teams, organisations (and their internal strata and divisions), and wider institutions (Bell *et al.* 2011). Patient safety is thus an example of the more general phenomenon known as the 'problem of many hands' (Thompson 1980). Described by the political philosopher Dennis Thompson, it applies to situations where many people contribute in many different ways to particular outcomes, so that the 'profusion of agents obscures the location of agency' (Thompson 2014: 1). Thompson offers two criteria that clarify individual moral responsibility in a collectivity:

1   the individual's actions or omissions make a causal contribution to the outcome and
2   these actions or omissions are not done in ignorance or under compulsion.

These criteria might best be understood as necessary but not sufficient conditions, such that individuals should be candidates for being held accountable for any actions or omissions only if they are met. In a healthcare context, a promising approach to augmenting these basic qualifying criteria is offered by the physician and ethicist Edmund Pellegrino (2004). Rejecting a no-blame system as a travesty of social and commutative justice, and emphasising the interdigitation and ethical reciprocity of individual and collective virtue, he proposes four major organising principles:

1   a properly organised organisational and systemic context is essential to reduce the prevalence of healthcare error;
2   its effectiveness and efficient working depend on a parallel affirmation of the moral duty and accountability of each health professional in the system;
3   each individual health professional must possess the competence and character crucial to the performance of her particular function as well as those of the system as a whole; and
4   the major function of a system is to reinforce and sustain these individual competencies and virtues.

For an accountability system to function, criteria and principles alone are not enough, however: also required is a structural arrangement that can make clear the relevant expectations and standards, define the actors that have responsibility for meeting those expectations and standards, create a forum to whom those actors are answerable, and enable the forum to pose questions, pass judgement, and impose consequences on the actors (Bovens 2007). We propose that, taken together, Thompson's criteria and Pellegrino's principles, along with an understanding of the structural requirements of an accountability system, provide a potentially useful framework for structuring thinking about questions of individual responsibility and its intersection with systems. Yet, as practice theory makes clear, such a framework is, by itself, likely to be sterile in the absence of empirical evidence. In this chapter, we use the framework as a starting point for analysis of the role of personal accountability for patient safety using ethnographic data from contrasting hospital contexts.

Methods

We conducted ethnographic case studies of five large acute hospitals (Table 1): two (Sukutra and Nikalele) in two low-income African countries and three (Farnchester, Greenborough and Worpford) in England, a high-income setting. These case studies were selected from

Table 1   *Details of the five ethnographic case studies*

Site	Interviews	Observations	Staff roles and areas of observation
Sukutra hospital Location: Africa Teaching, referral hospital	30 individuals	30 days (131 hours)	Physicians, nurses, midwives, clinical technicians, senior and middle managers, administrative staff. Surgical, neonatal, maternity services
Nikalele hospital Location: Africa Teaching, referral hospital	31 individuals	46 days (177 hours)	Physicians, nurses, midwives, clinical technicians, senior and middle managers, administrative staff. Surgical, neonatal, maternity services
Farnchester hospital Location: UK Teaching, referral hospital	32 individuals	41 days (252 hours)	Physicians, nurses, operating room and administrative staff, senior and middle managers. Surgical, neonatal, renal, infection prevention and control services and emergency departments.
Greenborough hospital Location: UK Teaching, referral hospital	13 individuals	6 days (38 hours)	Physicians, nurses, clinical technicians, senior and middle managers, administrative staff. Surgical, neonatal, infection prevention and control services.
Worpford hospital Location: UK Teaching, referral hospital	20 individuals	9 days (66 hours)	Physicians, nurses, ODPs, healthcare assistants, midwives, senior and middle managers. Surgical and maternity services.
Total:	126 individuals	132 days (664 hours)	

two research projects with similar aims and design. Four cases – two in England and two in Africa – were drawn from Project 1, which examined quality and safety in high and low-income countries. The data collected from the English sites was less extensive than from the African sites, so one case was augmented using data from its participation in Project 2, a study of culture and behaviour related to quality and safety in the English NHS (Dixon-Woods *et al.* 2013). A further English case was also selected from Project 2, yielding two African case studies and three UK case studies in total.

Ethical approval was obtained from each of the African sites and separately for the English sites. Further details are not provided in order to protect the anonymity of the sites. For the same reason, hospitals are given pseudonyms, and quotation labels give minimal identifying information (site and professional role). At the request of the research participants, the countries in which African sites were located have not been named. Thus, while we do not intend to imply an unwarranted degree of similarity across different African countries, we are restricted in the healthcare system details we can provide. What can be reported is that both African hospitals were government-run, teaching referral hospitals located in towns, serving a mixed urban-rural population. All three UK hospitals were large NHS teaching hospitals located in cities and serving as tertiary centres for a wider region.

With the verbal permission of staff and, where appropriate, that of patients, more than 660 hours of wide-ranging non-participation observation were undertaken in diverse areas of the five hospitals (76 days in Sukutra and Nikalele; 56 days in the English hospitals) covering managerial and clinical meetings as well as clinical activity. Interviews (some group-based) were conducted with informed consent from 124 hospital staff (Table 1) and were digitally recorded, translated where necessary and transcribed verbatim. At the interviewees' request, two other interviews were not recorded; notes were taken instead. Recruitment of participants was guided by purposive sampling to ensure diversity in terms of seniority, role, profession, subspecialty and area of practice. Interview topics covered perceptions of influences on and challenges of achieving patient safety.

Analysis of data was based on the constant comparative method (Charmaz 2006), which was informed, but not constrained, by sensitising constructs derived from the research questions and the relevant literature. The initial framework (based on Pellegrino and Thompson) proved very useful for structuring thinking about accountabilities of individuals and systems, but also required modification in light of the empirical findings. Supported by NVIVO software (QSR International, Brisbane), ELA led the analysis of data, including development of a coding scheme applied across all transcripts. MDW and MP reviewed samples of coded extracts at different stages and helped to refine analytic categories. By comparing and contrasting cases from diverse contexts, we sought to move beyond description of differences to theoretical insights (Druckman 2005). Conducting this kind of analysis involves multiple sensitivities, especially when it involves such diverse contexts of resources, history and environments. In order to avoid pathologising any particular setting or group, it is important to stress that our findings should not be read as the essentialist traits of any particular society, country or professional grouping.

Findings

Our observations and interviews across the five sites repeatedly confirmed the collective nature of the healthcare enterprise and the extent to which patient safety depended on contributions from many hands. For patients to remain safe, multiple interacting microsystems – from equipment design, maintenance and supply through administrative procedures to the performance of clinical practices, and much else – needed to go right. The extreme interdependence of each individual upon others meant that the individual who was most proximal to a specific poor outcome or 'near miss' was only rarely solely responsible. (For example, on one occasion it was observed that a nurse in Sukutra had forgotten to administer prophylactic antibiotics before surgery; however, as we go on to show, such errors were arguably a reflection of more systemic challenges within the organisational context.) But rarely too was their contribution completely negligible, and sometimes a particular individual's efforts were essential to preventing harm (for example, a neonatal nurse in an English site raising the alarm about monitoring equipment that did not appear to be functioning properly). Further, we found that an approach that focused solely on specific incidents or events offered only a partial and misleading account; consistent with practice theory, individuals also contributed to the prevailing conditions and environments for safety through the norms they produced and reproduced and through their behaviours and demonstration of professional virtues. Thompson's criterion that individuals should make a causal contribution to safety was thus easily met much of the time, though the extent to which any individual was the single or most important cause was highly variable.

Thompson (1980: 909) emphasises that individuals cannot be accountable for actions and omissions done in 'ignorance', including 'the formal and informal expectations of the individual's official role'. But across the five hospitals, we found that the standards that individuals should meet – whether of practice or conduct – were not always clear to them, that official standards were heavily distorted by customary practice, and that multiple and sometimes competing conceptions of safe practice were in play. As Giddens anticipated, formal guidance played an ambivalent and unstable role as a source of standards for practice. One basic but pervasive problem concerned workers' awareness of the relevant rules. In the African hospitals, clinical and administrative protocols were often lacking entirely (though more were gradually being introduced) or workers lacked knowledge of those that did exist because they had not been trained. Most clinical areas lacked protocols for appropriate antibiotic prescribing, for example, although in one site work was being undertaken with outside experts to develop local protocols for the neonatal and surgery departments. In the English hospitals, the problem was not so much too few protocols as too many, and policies that changed too frequently: workers reported that it was simply impossible to keep up to date, partly because of cuts to training:

> That induction part is not there, you will just be employed and you will be assigned to one ward and you start working with the people there. [Manager, Nikele]

> Six months down the line the staff that needed educating haven't been taught what they needed to know. [Manager, Worpford]

The challenges of making clear to people what was expected of them went well beyond formal standards, however. What individuals saw themselves as responsible for was profoundly shaped both by organisational contexts – which were typically rich in operational and managerial defects – and by the prevailing cultural norms. Workers frequently identified gaps between what they were supposed to do and the available resources for achieving it, pointing to problems with equipment, staffing, infrastructure and management as well as poorly designed and poorly functioning micro-systems (Aveling et al. 2015). Though the material deprivations were far more pronounced in the African sites, the nature of the pressures was often strikingly similar, such that the differences were of degree rather than of kind:

> Sometimes you don't find anaesthetic drugs, sometimes you don't find stitches, sometimes you don't find oxygen, sometimes you don't find gloves. [Doctor, Sukutra]

> They need to intubate a child, but they've only got one laryngoscope and it's not a small one suitable for children. The senior anaesthetist says 'you see? … that's what happens here, this is ridiculous. Apparently we're supposed to make do'. [Observation, Farnchester]

Pellegrino's stipulation that an organisational and systemic context supportive of safety should exist was therefore frequently violated. One response to these challenges involved individuals in seizing and exercising responsibility. We routinely witnessed staff keeping patients safe in the face of organisational failings by working extremely hard, finding creative solutions or 'working around' defects. For example, neonatal units in the African sites frequently lacked sufficient continuous positive airway pressure (CPAP) machines for the number of infants who needed breathing assistance; on their own initiative, local staff had fashioned home-made devices. In English neonatal units, nurses reported informally re-organising their work to compensate for the gaps when staff shortages occurred:

> You should always do hourly [observations] and generally we're quite good at working as a team so that if you're busy and you don't get to do it then somebody will come and do it for you […] there's been cases in the past where we' ve been ridiculously busy and somebody has sorted somebody else's patient. [Nurse, Greenborough]

These and other examples are, as Pellegrino suggests, illustrations of how the moral agency of individuals may be required to maintain the border between preventable and non-preventable harm. But sometimes the norms of practice were not so supportive of safety. The adverse nature of the environments in which people worked and the sheer volume of hazards that had to be negotiated had generalised effects, leaving many staff feeling overwhelmed, depleted and demoralised:

> 'Pray for me that I can find another job and leave this place', said one of the nurses. [Observation, Nikalele]

> The nurses talked about how this was really not what they signed up for. They talked about getting other jobs in shops. [Observation, Farnchester]

Staff felt deprived of control and, accordingly, perceived that their agency was limited. On occasion, this meant that they did not appear to accept or to exercise personal responsibility, even when to do so seemed possible and might have secured a better experience or outcomes for the patient. For instance a frail, elderly patient who fell partially out of bed in an English hospital was left hanging in some distress for several minutes while staff nearby completed cleaning another bed, despite being made aware of the situation. In one of the African hospitals, administration of fluids and antibiotics to a very sick baby was delayed by several hours. When a senior doctor asked a junior doctor why this had happened, the junior doctor at first replied that the parents had not brought the drugs, then that the drugs were out-of-stock. A few minutes of investigation by the senior doctor found the drugs nearby. The junior had put little effort into finding them, and then given excuses: his sense of personal responsibility was conditioned by a norm that 'nothing is ever available here'. In the African sites, students and trainees sometimes attempted tasks well beyond the limits of their competence, either in order to gain experience or because no-one else was available, and they sometimes made serious errors that harmed patients.

These examples appear to stumble on Pellegrino's requirement that each individual health professional must possess the competence and character crucial to the performance of her particular function. But they also show that local norms did not reinforce and sustain these individual competencies and virtue, suggesting that the conduct and behaviour of any individual needs to be understood in its social context. Importantly, these local norms were profoundly (though not exclusively) shaped by the wider socio-material, economic and historical context. For example, in all hospitals staff-to-patient ratios were repeatedly identified as the most important influence on quality and safety, but they were rarely within the control of individual units or even hospital administrators because of externally-set funding levels and the restricted availability of trained healthcare workers.

In the African hospitals, apparently invincible material deprivations, a sense that access to any care (regardless of its quality) was an improvement, and a background context of high (albeit improving) rates of infant mortality and tragic historical events also influenced normative expectations of standards of care. Thus, death and suffering were sometimes seen as normal and unavoidable, and the space for feasible action – and personal responsibility – accordingly shrunk:

> I say [to doctor], 'I'm sorry to hear you have had a few deaths this week' and he said 'yes, but they were all already very poor prognosis babies'. Basically he was saying they weren't avoidable. But some visiting doctors who were working in the unit at the time told me they felt there were in fact avoidable deaths (e.g. one baby died after being in an incubator that wasn't switched on). [Observation, Nikalele]

The deeply ingrained nature of guiding norms meant that some actions and omissions were not readily visible to some staff as violations of standards for which they should have to account. A rather different problem arose when staff felt that they had little choice about their actions, even when they knew the right thing to do. Much concern was reported by participants about the fairness of devolving blame to specific teams and individuals when the problems were felt to originate in external contexts over which they had no control. Several African senior managers, for example, protested that their hospitals were not responsible for failings of care when the reasons for those failings – including a refusal to appoint more staff or to allow patient admissions to be limited – lay with regional or national level authorities. Managers in the English hospitals similarly protested that they were constantly forced to function within externally imposed restrictions, targets, and processes that frustrated rather than assisted them in creating the conditions of safety (McKee *et al.* 2013).

> I don't think anybody has the right to penalise us. [Senior manager, Sukutra]

> There are many deaths, every day death, and every day it is really hurting. We receive children in numbers beyond our capacity. If the Director does not decide to limit [the number of admissions] when we have exhausted our capacity, what can we do? [Nurse, Nikalele]

> I asked can you talk to anybody about that [staffing levels] and she said she could tell the nurse manager but it just goes nowhere. She said the powers that be just don't listen. [Observation, Farnchester]

For workers at all levels, externally-imposed deprivations of control contributed to a feeling of restricted autonomy and a pervasive sense that it was unreasonable and unfair to hold individuals personally to account. This was a highly consequential problem because, as Pellegrino specifies, affirmation of the moral duty and accountability of each individual in the system is important to patient safety.

All five sites did feature forums which, in principle at least, could call individuals to account, pose questions and pass judgement (Bovens 2007). They were of multiple types, both internal and external to organisations, and were of varying degrees of formality – ranging from peers and colleagues through to external bodies with formal duties of oversight. Some of these external accountability forums, including regulators or accreditation agencies with powers to set standards, inspect, and take action, were of fairly recent origin, particularly in the African sites.

Positive effects of such forums were evident throughout our case studies. Externally-set standards, targets or goals were sometimes important in helping to remake norms about what was acceptable and to mobilise organisational commitment, largely by setting clear and explicit standards and then holding organisations to account for meeting them. In the English hospitals, these effects were clearly seen, for example, in relation to healthcare-associated infections:

> They started to gradually release Department of Health documents and guidance that was meant to drive organisations to improve standards … the Health and Social Care Act is a must-do, because it's an Act of Parliament and [organisations] can be legislatively penalised so that really governs the work that we do. [Infection control manager, Farnchester]

The need to account externally not only mobilised changes in organisational procedures, it also helped to signal and reinforce organisational and professional norms by motivating those at the senior levels of hierarchies to take action. For instance, in the African hospitals, a new accreditation requirement to hold and record regular morbidity and mortality (M&M) meetings gave impetus and standing to forums that held individuals to account for standards of professional integrity and competence. At one African M&M meeting, a case concerned twin babies who died because of failures to recognise and act on signs of worsening sepsis caused by the illegitimate absence of a doctor from scheduled duty. In this case, the senior doctor leading the meeting declined to attribute blame to the system, identifying it instead as a lapse in professional duty and thus as one of Bosk's unforgivable errors:

> The local senior doctor says 'so the issue is the doctor who did not round on Sunday. Diseases don't go to pray on Sunday do they? The doctor on duty was not there to do the ward round'. He then adds that 'you need to do your part. The system may have problems, but you must do your part'. [Observation, Nikalele]

We also found, however, that the available accountability forums – whether internal or external – did not always support the positive affirmations of individuals' duties and accountabilities. The different forums sometimes competed, conflicted, failed to cohere or gave rise to underlaps and overlaps. Whatever form they took, these forums sometimes tolerated poor practice and conduct when they lacked the authority, will, or capacity to act. These failures often occurred at the managerial level:

At the moment there is no follow up … so I can create an action plan but no-one other than me will take responsibility for coming back and saying well did you achieve what you said you would? [Nurse manager, Worpford]

When forums were absent or failed to impose consequences, some aspects of care tended over time to become normed as optional or to be sloppily performed. For instance, use of a surgical safety checklist was mandated in England by the government in the UK and by the accreditation frameworks used in the African countries. In one African site, the absence of a forum responsible for monitoring its use and the inability of individual nurses to challenge (high status) physicians meant that sanctions for non-use or poor use were not applied. Ultimately the site abandoned the checklist altogether.

In all settings, forums that might have promoted individual accountability were thwarted because career development and job security depended crucially upon maintaining relationships with senior figures, often creating oppressive conditions where individuals were fearful of the personal consequences of any attempts to 'speak up' to superiors or challenge peers about their concerns. Managers in all settings reported that they often felt limited in their power to discipline or control clinical staff – especially senior physicians. In part, this was because of lack of leadership capacity, but it was also linked to the dependence of managers on the cooperation of those they seek to manage (Harvey *et al.* 2014). In the African hospitals, managerial willingness to take unpopular action against highly-qualified staff was further undermined by the ability of such staff to move elsewhere given skill shortages nationally. Medical students and trainees – who provided most of the day-to-day medical care – were accountable to senior, fully qualified doctors, yet those senior doctors were only rarely present in clinical areas. Students and trainees did not always demonstrate the competence or character necessary to secure the safety of their patients, but – in contrast to the sanctioning behaviours of the attending physicians in *Forgive and Remember* and in contradiction of Pellegrino's requirements – the system did not reinforce nor sustain these individual competencies and virtues:

Students are doing the cases that should be done by seniors in this hospital. Then afterwards, patients develop infections. When this happens, there is no one that questions the doer. There is no accountability. [Midwife, Sukutra]

In one African site, the institutional arrangements for accountability were especially problematic. Here, the university ran the hospital. Employed by or educationally dependent on the university, physicians and students were accountable to the university, not the hospital's management. One consequence was that training needs were routinely prioritised over patient care and safety. This was evident in the persistent over-crowding of clinical areas by students, which made it difficult to perform procedures safely, control infection, or respect patients' privacy. Midwives, nurses and others who protested found it difficult to secure cooperation because they could not call students to account, and thus could not function as a forum:

When one mother delivers there are a lot of people who stand there and attend … Students from all batches attend. When you tell them to leave the ward, they refuse. [Midwife, Sukutra]

In principle the exercise of personal moral responsibility might resolve the problem; students could simply vacate crowded spaces or organise themselves to attend in smaller groups. That they did not do so might be seen as 'weakness of the will' (Akrasia), but perhaps is better treated as evidence of how behaviours were institutionally organised and structured by the opportunities provided to individuals to be 'good': the organisation did not provide alternative ways of being educated, and the behaviour was heavily normed. In Pellegrino's terms, this amounts to a failure to cultivate the conditions of virtuous conduct amounting to constraints on choice of action, but Pellegrino would not rule out a role for personal responsibility altogether. Indeed, sufficient individuals choosing a more virtuous path might be enough to reform the norm, so that a collectivity would act back on the system and in so doing provoke change.

We also found that some accountability forums had negative effects, particularly when the environment was excessively harsh and punitive, when the consequences seemed arbitrary or applied to the wrong parties, and when norms of justice and fairness were violated. Across all hospitals, participants reported didactic, authoritarian, and sometimes aggressive, bullying behaviour by senior colleagues that blamed individuals for problems over which they had little control:

> At the end of the case presentation the senior doctor says 'do you have any questions? What have we discussed?! Eh? Eh?! (aggressive voice). If you've learned nothing then go to the streets!' [Observation, Nikalele]

> Bullying is probably the right word actually, there's a big network of very very senior managers that are just driven about targets. [Nurse manager, Greenborough]

Individuals often lacked confidence that there would be some predictable and fairly applied due process in the event of something going wrong. In African sites, participants reported concerns that incidents would be investigated by agencies lacking the necessary knowledge and skills (e.g. the police). Again consistent with Giddens's argument about the triumph of local norms over external rules and mandates, participants in all sites feared that much of the real power lay outside the formal structure, and that informal consequences frustrated the operation of the formal processes and procedures or (at a minimum) undermined their purpose:

> I have talked to someone [who tried to take disciplinary action], there was a sort of harassment directed towards him. At the end of the day you are an individual […] if you have somebody who is dependent on you, it's very difficult to go ahead with such type of confrontation. [Doctor, Sukutra]

> You only have to look around where any organisation in the NHS will hound whistleblowers, because they make the organisation look bad […] and if staff put their heads above the parapet and start to try and make a noise and say 'we're concerned', they get their heads blown off. [Doctor, Greenborough]

The sense of vulnerability was exacerbated by lack of confidence in the transparency, predictability and fairness of processes associated with patient complaints. In African hospitals, staff particularly feared intimidation by patients' families, unjust or corrupt prosecutions, and lack of access to legal advice or poor support from their employers:

> Corruption is the commonest problem everywhere, be it legal system or medical system, it's everywhere. [Doctor, Sukutra]

Because students and trainees in the African hospitals feared being humiliated, suffering educational penalties at the hands of their superiors, or being drawn into potentially corrupt or non-transparent legal actions, they were sometimes reluctant to acknowledge errors and failures of care both in documentation and when reporting to seniors. As a result, what they reported or documented in patient records was not always what had actually happened. In UK sites, while staff had more confidence in the predictability and resources for medico-legal procedures, some nonetheless reported that fears of being bullied and of damage to their career prospects inhibited their giving voice to safety concerns.

Discussion and conclusions

Our analysis provides empirical support for understanding patient safety both as contingent on the dynamic, emergent and recursive duality of structure and agency in healthcare settings and as the outcome of collective effort. It shows, consistent with practice theory, that each individual in a healthcare system typically makes a causal contribution (however small) to outcomes, at the same time as the system shapes and structures the possibilities open to individuals. Across the five sites in our study, the availability of logistical support and resources and the prevailing cultural discourses or norms promoted, enabled or discouraged certain behaviours and practices in particular settings. In consequence, systems and individuals co-constructed the conditions of safety; each element acted on the other and was mutually constitutive. Our work affirms the ethical principle that individual moral responsibility for actions and behaviours is an irreducible element of professional practice, but also shows empirically that opportunities to 'be good' are institutionally organised and structured and that individuals make a crucial contribution towards the creation and reproduction of the normative conditions and criteria to by which they and their actions are to be held account. Without individuals assuming personal moral responsibility and exercising agency, getting the work done in healthcare and getting it done safely both become impossible. We propose the system/individual distinction that has dominated debates about patient safety is in fact a reification: individuals are not somehow 'outside' and separate from the system, since they create, modify and are subject to the social forces that are an inescapable feature of any organisational system.

Some safety problems in our case studies were examples of straightforward moral failings, and these actions or omissions by individuals – such as illegitimate absence from scheduled duty – were blameworthy. As both Thompson and Pellegrino make clear, such culpable failures cannot be justified by reference to the context, notwithstanding the evident challenges of those contexts. And, as Bosk argues, in such instances the exercise of social control through sanctions and other means of reinforcing professional norms is essential to protecting patients from potential harm in the long-run as well as to the maintenance of professional community. At the other end of the spectrum, situations where there was no scope for personal responsibility were also generally clear and unambiguous. Much more common were situations where some space – albeit protean in form – for personal responsibility remained: the interdependence of individual behaviours and organisational and systemic contexts was repeatedly evidenced. Individuals often triumphed in the face of adversity through the exercise of a morally-founded agency. Where apparently unjustified failures to act on moral responsibility occurred, it seemed that the conscious choices and actions of individuals were heavily conditioned by strongly reinforced norms and other constraints, some of them deeply institutionally and historically patterned.

Participants at all levels of organisational hierarchies were frequently working in settings that not only failed to enable them to provide safe care but also failed to cultivate the conditions of virtuous conduct. Patterned norms and routines acted as signals of what was acceptable practice. As we argued earlier, an important consequence of this is that the perceptions of local actors may be an unreliable guide to questions of moral responsibility or the moral content of actions or omissions: the most insidious form of power 'consists of letting people whose business it is define what that business includes, which versions of it are serious and important, and which don't matter much.' (Becker 1995: 307). Deeply institutionalised norms and routinised forms of justification may be used both to promote excellent care and to legitimate or obscure poor practices that can harm patients (Dixon-Woods 2010). Many norms of acceptability and excusability were functional for hard-working and over-stretched staff (Dixon-Woods *et al.* 2009), but they were also sometimes implicated in allowing staff to externalise blame and to attenuate personal responsibility. Some norms rendered some problems – such as harm and assaults on dignity – as normal, natural troubles that were either invisible or inescapable given the circumstances of provision (Dixon-Woods *et al.* 2011). This in turn had the effect of depressing aspirations and normalising low expectations for quality of care, so that opportunities to improve care even when it was possible to do so were neglected. These findings illustrate the value of a more formal, principles-based framework for adjudicating on matters of personal responsibility and accountability in order to avoid a descent into unhelpful relativism. But they also underline how each individual contributes to the reproduction of norms about acceptable practice and the important responsibilities associated with that.

Importantly, this principle applies to every individual in an organisation, from the blunt end to the sharp end. Those at management and leadership level have moral agency and moral responsibility but, importantly, they may be subject to the same supports and inhibitors as those on the shop-floor. But an emphasis on the personal responsibility of managers and senior figures (internal and external to organisations) is needed to avoid bracketing these individuals as somehow part of 'the system' or and to avoid seeing patient safety as the sole responsibility of those at the sharp end. This is especially true given that some people are much more in a position to help cultivate the virtues of others; they may, for example, set the moral tone, model the values, or create and operate accountability processes. Thus, when organisations are not able to increase resources, leaders and managers retain an important role in setting and maintaining expectations of what can be done within the practical limits and providing the context in which the relevant professional virtues can be exercised.

A similar argument might be made in relation to formal standards of practice. If actors are to be made accountable, then the standards they need to meet must be defined and they must be aware of their responsibilities for meeting them. Yet we found workers were not always aware of the relevant standards. As Thompson (2014) notes, ignorance counts as an excuse only if the ignorance is not negligent. Across the five hospitals, lack of awareness was often organisationally induced, and might properly be understood as failures of organisations to provide clarity and enable or support compliance. In many such circumstances, holding individuals to account would not be fair, ethical or effective. But in other instances, it would be reasonable to require individuals to know what they did not know, and that they should not, for example, attempt complex surgery beyond the limits of their competence. This too relies on the clear articulation of standards, expectations and priorities, the consistent evidencing of these in organisational routines and practices, proper attention to them by organisational actors, and oversight by accountability forums.

Our findings suggest that accountability forums (both formal and informal) have the potential, as Pellegrino emphasises and Thompson implies, to improve systems and to influence norms of 'good' behaviour. We observed several encouraging examples of such forums, for example when they renewed or created understandings of the proper standards of care and of professional integrity and moral responsibility. Yet these effects were rarely straightforward or easy to achieve, and the forums often failed or had perverse effects. Accountability forums sometimes failed altogether because of weaknesses in leadership or capacity or because informal social systems and quasi-autonomous professional groups subverted formal systems. Thus, some morally culpable failures escaped with impunity and further reinforced unhelpful norms. Second, individuals feared that due process would not be served, that they would be blamed unfairly and unpredictably (for example for systems problems outside their control) and that the consequences imposed would be harsh and arbitrary. And some accountability forums faltered because many features of standards and answerability were not codified in the mechanisms and processes of accountability systems.

The normative, interpretive work entailed in calling to account was influenced by interrelated material, institutional and symbolic contexts. Thus, when forums sought to impose accountability frameworks underpinned by values of learning and improvement in contexts characterised by authoritarianism or punitive responses to errors, the clash of values created confusion of purpose. This, together with overwhelming structural constraints, weak systems for control and oversight, perceptions of corruption and nepotism in some contexts, and absence of follow-through when problems were detected, fuelled apathy and fatalism. The effect was to continually erode the morale, energy and will of staff and the distinction between genuinely insurmountable problems and less legitimate excuses.

Our analysis demonstrates the need to be sensitive to wider institutional contexts beyond both specific organisations and beyond healthcare. Many constraints on organisations and individuals arose institutionally. Individual organisations were rarely fully in control of their own destiny: budgets, resources, targets and policies were often externally imposed by regional or national government agencies. More broadly, in the African hospitals, the wider context undermined workers' beliefs that the legal systems and institutions of state would operate fairly and impartially, and that it was possible to survive personally by always acting in the collective interest.

Conclusions

These findings furnish empirical evidence of a basic sociological tenet of practice theory – the interdependence of systemic and individual agency at all levels – in the context of patient safety in healthcare systems. An uncritically-applied 'no blame' approach may fail to recognise variations in the type and scope of opportunities for individuals to assert their moral responsibility, but a calculus-like logic seeking to promote 'just culture' that fails to recognise the limits of individual autonomy and the messiness of standards of practice may be equally misguided. Individual agency is both an ethical requirement and a means of modifying systems themselves; never holding individuals to account risks normalisation of failure, fatalism, externalisation of blame and apathy, and may erode collective commitments and values. The ability to impose sanctions for culpable failures is likely to remain an important feature of any well-functioning accountability system, but legitimate and effective exercise of this ability depends on a predictable, fair and effectively operated institutional infrastructure, with proportionate consequences and alignment of the values and processes of different internal and external forums.

It is not a matter of balancing systems against individual accountability; instead, their recursive nature needs to be recognised. The opportunities for workers to 'be good' are made logistically possible and cultivated culturally both by the organisations they work in and by wider institutional structures. Accordingly, the interdependence of institutional and socio-material and economic contexts (within and beyond the hospital) needs to be taken into account in the design of accountability frameworks. Systems need to be designed and operated to support, cultivate and sustain individual competence and virtue, with explicit attention to how they encourage the norms and values that shape the exercise of moral agency. We conclude that an important responsibility both of organisations and accountability systems is the cultivation and enabling of individuals' moral agency and the fostering of the conditions of moral community. Making accountability 'work' for patient safety is not simply a question of designing the perfect algorithm for blame distribution; one of the major obligations of healthcare organisations (and wider institutions) in relation to patient safety is to nurture the conditions of moral community. Achieving this will require deep understanding of processes of social control.

Acknowledgements

We are grateful for the participation of the hospitals and staff involved in this study. We also thank Sophie Wilson for her help with coding of the data, and Janet Willars, Joel Minion, Graham Martin, Piotr Ozieranski, Ansha Nega and Yvette Kayonga for their help with data collection. This research was supported by the Wellcome Trust (WT097899M.) Some of the data reported here was collected as part of a project commissioned and funded by the Policy Research Programme (Reference No 0770017) in the Department of Health. The views expressed are not necessarily those of the Department. We are grateful to co-investigators and colleagues on this grant. MP's work in global health ethics is supported by a Wellcome Trust Strategic Award (096527). We thank Alan Cribb for invaluable comments on an earlier draft.

References

Aveling, E.L., Kayonga, Y., Nega, A. and Dixon-Woods, M. (2015) Why is patient safety so hard in low-income countries? A qualitative study of healthcare workers' views in two African hospitals, *Globalization and Health*, 11, 6.

Becker, H.S. (1995) The power of inertia, *Qualitative Sociology*, 18, 3, 301–9.

Bell, S.K., Delbanco, T., Anderson-Shaw, L., McDonald, T.B., *et al.* (2011) Accountability for medical error moving beyond blame to advocacy, *Chest*, 140, 2, 519–26.

Bosk, C.L. (2003) *Forgive and Remember: Managing Medical Failure*, 2nd edn. Chicago, IL: University of Chicago Press.

Bovens, M. (2007) Analysing and assessing accountability: A conceptual Framework1, *European Law Journal*, 13, 4, 447–68.

Brint, S. (2006) Saving the 'soul of professions': Freidson's institutional ethics and the defence of professional autonomy, *Knowledge, Work and Society*, 4, 2, 101 –29.

Charmaz, K. (2006) *Constructing Grounded Theory: A Practical Guide through Qualitative Analysis*. London: Sage.

Dekker, S. (2012) *Just culture: Balancing safety and accountability*. Ashgate Publishing.

Dixon-Woods, M. (2010) Why is patient safety so hard? A selective review of ethnographic studies, *Journal of Health Services Research & Policy*, 15, Suppl 1, 11–6.

Dixon-Woods, M., Suokas, A., Pitchforth, E. and Tarrant, C. (2009) An ethnographic study of classifying and accounting for risk at the sharp end of medical wards, *Social Science & Medicine*, 69, 3, 362–9.

Dixon-Woods, M., Bosk, C.L., Aveling, E.L., Goeschel, C.A., *et al.* (2011) Explaining Michigan: Developing an ex post theory of a quality improvement program, *The Milbank Quarterly*, 89, 2, 167–205.

Dixon-Woods, M., Baker, M., Charles, J., Dawson, J., *et al.* (2013) Culture and behaviour in the english national health services: Overview of lessons from a large multi-method study, *BMJ Quality and Safety*, 23, 2, 106–15.

Druckman, D. (2005) Comparative case study approaches. In Druckman, D. (ed.), *Doing Research*. Oakland, CA: Sage.

Feldman, M.S. and Orlikowski, W.J. (2011) Theorizing practice and practicing theory, *Organization Science*, 22, 5, 1240–53.

Freidson, E. (2001) *Professionalism: The Third Logic*. Cambridge: Polity Press.

Giddens, A. (1984) *The Constitution of Society: Outline of the Theory of Structuration*. Berkeley, CA: University of California Press.

Harvey, J., Annandale, E., Loan-Clarke, J., Suhomlinova, O., *et al.* (2014) Mobilising identities: The shape and realities of middle and junior managers' working lives – a qualitative study, *Health Services and Delivery Research*, 2, 11.

Kant, I. (1973) *Critique of Pure Reason*. London: Macmillan.

Kohn, L.T., Corrigan, J. and Donaldson, M.S. (2000) *To Err is Human: Building a Safer Health System*. Joseph Henry Press.

Leape, L.L., Kabcenell, A.I., Gandhi, T.K., Carver, P., *et al.* (2000) Reducing adverse drug events: Lessons from a breakthrough series collaborative, *Joint Commission Journal on Quality and Patient Safety*, 26, 6, 321–31.

Marx, D. (2001) Patient safety and the 'just culture': A primer for health care executives. Prepared for Columbia University Under Flagrant Provided by the National Heart, Lung, and Blood Institute. Available at: Www.Mers-Tm.net/support/marx_primer.Pdf. Date last accessed 23 April 2015.

McKee, L., Charles, K., Dixon-Woods, M., Willars, J., *et al.* (2013) New and distributed leadership in quality and safety in healthcare, or 'old' and hierarchical? An interview study with strategic stakeholders, *Journal of Health Services Research and Policy*, 18, Suppl 2, 11–9.

Meadows, S., Baker, K. and Butler, J. (2005) The incident decision tree, *Clinical Risk*, 11, 2, 66–8.

Pellegrino, E.D. (2002) Professionalism, profession and the virtues of the good physician, *Mount Sinai Journal of Medicine*, 69, 6, 378–84.

Pellegrino, E.D. (2004) Prevention of medical error: Where professional and organizational ethics meet. *Accountability: Patient Safety and Policy Reform*. Washington, DC: Georgetown University Press, Washington.

Thompson, D.F. (1980) Moral responsibility of public officials: The problem of many hands, *The American Political Science Review*, 74, 4, 905–16.

Thompson, D.F. (2014) Responsibility for failures of government the problem of many hands, *The American Review of Public Administration*, 44, 3, 259–73.

Wachter, R.M. (2013) Personal accountability in healthcare: Searching for the right balance, *BMJ Quality & Safety*, 22, 2, 176–80.

Wachter, R.M. and Pronovost, P.J. (2009) Balancing 'no blame' with accountability in patient safety, *New England Journal of Medicine*, 361, 14, 1401–6.

4

Enacting corporate governance of healthcare safety and quality: a dramaturgy of hospital boards in England

Tim Freeman, Ross Millar, Russell Mannion and Huw Davies

Introduction

Patient safety remains a high-profile health policy issue, traceable internationally since land-mark publications in the USA (Institute of Medicine 1999) and UK (Department of Health 2000) highlighted the scale of medical error and harm to patients. Errors were framed as con-ditioned, precipitated and exacerbated by systemic and latent organisational factors – and thus amenable to prevention (Waring *et al.* 2010). Empirical research informed by organi-sational psychology located clinical failures within organisational contexts ('clinical micro-systems'), seeing errors as the result of embedded unsafe practices rather than individual failings (Nelson *et al.* 2008). The solution proposed for this framing of the problem was implementation of standardised processes and 'designing out' errors, both at the level of specific interventions and whole-organisation safety systems. While this perspective informs much empirical patient safety research, Lamont and Waring (2015) offer a subtle reading of a tension evident within the literature: is patient safety a 'thing' that may be enhanced through technical solutions; or a more nebulous, contested phenomenon requiring attendance to the socio-cultural context of proposed changes to practice (Rowley and Waring 2011)? From a socio-cultural perspective, transfer of technical 'solutions' between industries risks subver-sion by existing professional hierarchies, as observed by Currie *et al.* (2009) in an evaluation of incident reporting techniques developed in the aviation industry and subsequently imple-mented within a hospital. Crucially, it is feared that embedded social and organisational prac-tices which make technical systems work within their original contexts may be overlooked (Macrae 2014); and that this explains the limited impact of patient safety interventions (Sheldon *et al.* 2004). The implication is that greater attention is required to ambiguities at play, and greater insight into the lived experience of patient safety work requires combination of theory with empirical data.

The failure of the Executive board to ensure safe clinical practice was implicated in events at Mid Staffordshire NHS Trust in the UK (Francis 2013) where many patients received sub-standard care in a context of chaotic management systems. The detailed response to these events is outlined in *A promise to learn – a commitment to act* (Department of Health 2013) which informed development of a National Patient Safety Alert System, publication of 'never events' data, and a Patient Safety Collaboratives programme to support improvements. As entities with statutory responsibilities for oversight, boards have ultimate responsibility for upholding the quality and safety of care delivered within their organisation, and are

The Sociology of Healthcare Safety and Quality, First Edition. Edited by Davina Allen, Jeffrey Braithwaite, Jane Sandall and Justin Waring. Chapters © 2016 The Authors. Book Compilation © 2016 Foundation for the Sociology of Health & Illness/Blackwell Publishing Ltd.

charged with a fundamental role in the governance of patient safety through defining and managing objectives, strategy, priorities, culture and systems of organisational control (NHS Leadership Academy 2013).

Empirical literature identifies governance practices as potentially important in safeguarding patient safety, including routine feedback and monitoring of statistical data, strategic involvement of clinicians in quality improvement, and attention to external governance systems (Jha and Epstein 2010, Jiang *et al.* 2009, 2011, Vaughn *et al.* 2006). However, as with the broader patient safety research literature above, considerable weaknesses in study design and theoretical orientation remain (Millar *et al.* 2013). While qualitative and case-study research is emerging (Baker *et al.* 2010, Ramsay *et al.* 2010), significant gaps remain in our understanding of the processes of organisation associated with board governance of patient safety in hospital settings (Chambers and Cornforth 2012). Specifically, we lack detailed understanding of what board members do, and the manner in which they do so, as they seek to discharge obligations with regard to patient safety (Millar *et al.* 2013, Nicolini *et al.* 2011, Waring 2007). The concept performativity may prove helpful in exploring board practices (Freeman and Peck 2007, 2010), the purpose of this chapter being to explore its application empirically.

Below, we introduce performativity and consider its influence within the study of organisational life; trace its foundations to the work of Austin (1962) and Goffman (1974); and note its empirical application in the context of participatory governance (Hajer 2004). We then employ Hajer's framework of scripting, setting, staging and performance to hospital executive board meetings, and explore implications for patient safety governance.

The foundations of performativity: Austin and Goffman

Austin (1962) coined the neologism 'performativity' to describe instances in which the utterance of a phrase constitutes an action which changes reality rather than describes it; a simultaneous 'saying' and 'doing' which requires others to act in accordance with its implications. Austin's paradigmatic case is the phrase 'I do' when spoken within the context of a marriage ceremony; a phrase requiring those exchanging vows to act, and be acted upon by others, as a married couple from that point forward. Austin additionally stipulates that performative utterances are meaningful actions that are neither true nor false but generative, that is, they create a social reality.

While Austin defines performativity, Goffman's (1974) dramaturgy of social interactions applies a theatrical metaphor to indirectly explore its operation, principally through framing. For Goffman, the framing of the stage – the separation of front of stage, backstage and audience, and reciprocal acceptance of the roles of audience and players – shapes the performativity of utterances onstage. In an extension of earlier work on the presentation of self (Goffman 1959), Goffman notes that performativities are made possible through framing. Frames are essentially classification systems which actors use to order and make sense of diverse social phenomena, so that the performative potential of an utterance depends upon the frames available.

The rise of 'performativity'

From its inception within linguistic philosophy (Austin 1962), the reach of performativity has ballooned. Early areas of influence include theoretical development in the emergence of order in complex interactive systems (Bateson 1972); the framing, staging and (re)creation of social life (Goffman 1974); and the 'language games' structuring performative utterances (Lyotard 1979). Later applications include the constitution of gendered identity through interactions (Butler 1993, 2010); the continuous (re)construction of society (Latour 1986, 1987); and the effects of economic theory upon action (Callon 1998). Organisationally, performativity has informed analysis of continuous change present in the enactment of organisational routines (Feldman and Pentland 2003); the enactment of technology within social settings (Law and Singleton 2000, Orlikowski and Scott 2008); the role of storytelling in coordinating within and between organisations (Diedrich *et al.* 2011); and organisational change as active translation rather than passive diffusion (Czarniawska and Sevon 1996).

The performativity of governance: Hajer

Informed by Goffman's earlier work, Hajer (2005, Hajer and Versteeg 2005) provides a dramaturgical framework for analysing the performative dimensions of public governance through consideration of the setting(s) in which deliberation takes place and the enactment of organisational frames, operationalised through consideration of the scripting, setting, staging and performance of governance. Scripting refers to the determination of actors involved in the decision-making forum. Consistent with the generative potential of performativity it considers how participatory practices construct participants as either active or passive; collaborators or protesters; competent or incompetent. In contrast, setting concerns the physical environment of interaction, including artefacts (e.g. minutes of previous meetings) that participants bring to the physical environment and which shape performance. Deliberate attempts to organise interaction between participants is identified as staging. It is achieved by drawing on existing symbols, the invention of new ones, and conventions governing distinctions between active players and passive audiences; what might be termed 'unwritten rules of engagement'. The final category, performance, concerns interactions which (re)construct knowledge/power relationships that shape future interactions, providing opportunities for change over time.

If Goffman is correct that reality is mediated through the application of frames to make sense of available information, then all accounts of reality are shaped. The implication, in the context of patient safety governance, is that the examination of safety could be framed in many ways with radically different consequences for action. For example, in presenting data that indicates a breach of an infection control performance target, is this: an instance of unreliable data requiring a defence of organisational practice? Or a worrying event requiring detailed diagnostic work to uncover systemic problems and institute quality improvement activity? Or an impossibly harsh target imposed by regulators requiring robust challenge? We explore empirically the operation of such performativities in relation to the board governance of patient safety, applying Hajer's analytic framework to qualitative data collected through overt non-participant observation at four case-study sites within the English NHS.

Methods

Design
The overall study design is a comparative case study across multiple (n = 4) study sites (Stake 1995). Each case had at its centre an acute Foundation Trust (FT) hospital – an independent public benefit organisation based on mutual traditions subject to independent external regulation (NHS Leadership Academy 2013). Membership of FT management boards comprises a chair, chief executive, executive directors and independent (non-executive)

directors (NEDs) who are, with the chair, in the majority. All board members bear responsibility, individually and collectively, for performance and the quality of services (NHS Leadership Academy 2013).

Sample selection

Cases reflect the diversity of English NHS hospital FT trusts: a district general hospital; a teaching hospital with a global reputation for specialist services and innovation; a regional centre offering specialist services; and a trust undertaking large-scale service redesign. Further specific details, including cultural characteristics of board meetings, is provided in Table 1.

Cases were additionally selected on the basis of their performance trajectory over the last three years on a range of safety and quality indicators selected from the Dr. Foster database for 2011. Every year Dr. Foster publishes a Hospital Guide that uses publicly available statistics to measure and assess what is happening in hospitals in England to increase transparency in relation to variations in performance. The data focuses on indicators in three domains of quality obtained from the available statistics, combined with information from self-reporting

Table 1   *Summary of each case study site*

Arran	'World-class provider',
	• Global aspirations built on research & development
	• Strategic focus; external horizon-scanning to secure compliance with policy directives and safeguard the self-image of the trust as a pre-eminent provider.
	• Strong 'shaping' steer by the CEO: low challenge by non-execs and a strong medical executive team
	• Needing to address emerging performance issues while minimising damage to its 'world class' self-image
Skye	'Local service under pressure'
	• District general hospital trust (3 sites)
	• Rotating board membership for over 3 years.
	• A myriad of problems
	• Focus on internal problem solving, limited wider strategy
	• High internal challenge by non-execs, a strong chair, technocratic CEO finding his feet
Lewis	'Embattled regional powerhouse'
	• A large teaching hospital
	• Seen as the main regional provider
	• Dominant CEO acting as a political antagonist; defending local interests from competing regional and national forces
	• Estate, finance, and legal disputes
Islay	'Faith in quality improvement methodologies'
	• A district general hospital trust
	• An 'intelligent' board
	– Reasoned and assured questioning by non-execs;
	– CQI culture;
	– Emphasis on patient experience
	• Strategic focus
	– reconfiguration and integrated care strategies
	– Clinical oversight
	– divisions 'invited' to provide updates

of safety aspects from an annual questionnaire. We used these data to select two case study sites indicated as getting worse (in the light of overall improvement of other hospitals) and two that were improving. Trust sites have been anonymised by being renamed after Scottish islands; the two improving trusts are Islay and Arran, the two getting worse Lewis and Skye.

Data collection and analysis
Acting in pairs, the authors undertook overt non-participant observation of four sequential management board meetings at each case study site, totalling approximately 50 hours of observation. Of the major topic areas discussed, issues relating to service quality, patient safety, performance measurement, and risk formed a substantial part of board meeting time at each site (Table 2). The authors are all experienced social policy researchers with established interests in the governance of healthcare quality, and data collection was designed to facilitate an analysis of Hajer's analytic framework. Descriptive free-text field notes were taken by observers at each meeting, supplemented with documentary data including the agenda, supporting chapters and (retrospectively upon completion) minutes of each meeting. Data from field notes were compiled across multiple board meetings within each trust to detail board operations and identify the manner in which board governance of patient safety was enacted. We used the analytic dimensions of scripting, setting, staging and performance identified by Hajer (2005) as a deductive *a priori* template (code book) against which qualitative material were organised.

Thematic analysis revealed patterns (similarities and differences) within the data, showing the divergent dramaturgies at play within each specific site. While these enactments were found to be stable across multiple meetings within sites, they proved substantially different between sites.

Findings

We first outline the operation of the board at each site to retain the integrity of each organisational setting, then offer a comparative analysis of Hajer's dramaturgical categories 'scripting', 'setting' and 'staging' in sequence across sites, indicating the scope and scale of

Table 2   *Summary of board time by topic area across all four observed meetings*

Topic areas	Arran		Skye		Lewis		Islay	
	Mins	*(%)*	*Mins*	*(%)*	*Mins*	*(%)*	*Mins*	*(%)*
Service quality, patient safety, performance measurement, risk	252	(60)	379	(42)	236	(28)	448	(54)
Strategy and capacity	30	(7)	185	(21)	158	(19)	315	(38)
HR	56	(13)	79	(9)	13	(2)	31	(4)
Finance	83	(20)	55	(6)	105	(12)	28	(3)
Estates	–	–	–	–	198	(23)	8	(1)
Other	–	–	194	(22)	130	(17)	–	–
Total	421	(100)	892	(100)	845	(100)	830	(100)

The table summarises the amount of time spent in minutes (percentage of total time) on specific, frequently occurring, topic areas within each case study site, totalled across all of the four board meetings at each site. All board meetings devoted considerable time to issues of service quality, patient safety, performance measurement and risk, and this composite measure took the longest amount of time at each of the sites.

differences between sites (table 3). We then explore the final dramaturgical category, 'performance', in relation to board deliberation of indicators associated with infection control, a key component of the external performance management regime within the English NHS.

Site 1: Arran – a world-class provider

Arran has a strong research culture and global reputation for service innovation. The board acts strategically and is externally oriented, seeking to secure compliance with central policy directives while further developing its global reach and status as a pre-eminent provider and academic research centre. In operation, board meetings are highly formal and structured to enable the CEO to 'steer' interpretations of events. The executive team are experienced with low turnover and a strong medical presence. Non-executives exhibit low levels of challenge even when performance difficulties are under discussion; indeed, the dynamic of board meetings could be summarised as maintenance of the narrative of 'world class' status while engaging with potential performance difficulties evident in summary indicator data.

Site 2: Skye – a local service under pressure

In marked contrast, Skye exhibits high levels of executive turnover and overt recognition of multiple problems in service provision, focusing on internal problems rather than strategy. board meetings are steered strongly by the chair who dominated a newly appointed CEO; strong challenges from Non-executives are common including expressions of disappointment at poor service performance and support for executives considered high performing. During the period of observation one executive stepped down, replaced by a deputy who received similarly high levels of challenge. Board dynamics could be summarised as routine non-executive challenge with limited long-term strategic direction.

Site 3: Lewis – an embattled regional powerhouse

Protective of its reputation as a regional centre, board meetings are structured to ensure that issues considered to be of strategic importance receive due consideration, events considered as they unfold over successive meetings. The image revealed is that of a guardian of local and wider regional interests, requiring continued political influence. The executive team is experienced and longstanding and the CEO personifies the organisation, dominating board meetings and acting as a political antagonist to defend local interests. During observation considerable time was spent on a small number of financial and estate issues and related legal disputes considered strategically important. Non-executives were typically involved in clarifications related to their specific areas of interest rather than challenges over strategy or performance. Overall, the board dynamic could be characterised as one of defending 'regional champion' status.

Site 4: Islay – faith in quality improvement methodologies

The overwhelming impression of this site is one in which board structures and processes focus attention on reconfiguration and integrated care strategies. Central to this approach is the consideration of performance issues related to external regulatory requirements (infection control; pressure sores) directly linked to improvement work to support strategic plans. Patient experience is routinely invoked and normalised by the presentation of a patient experience narrative at the start of each board meeting. Non-executives are encouraged to question and their contributions are actively sought by the executive team. This board could be characterised as drawing on a wide range of soft and hard intelligence, seeking to maintain strategic focus while discharging external regulatory accountabilities.

Table 3 Summary of Hajer's dramaturgical categories by case study site

	Arran	Skye	Lewis	Islay
Scripting	CEO shaped events through 'CEO Report' agenda item; Low levels of Non-exec challenge; Opportunities to challenge 'managed'	chair dominant; Non-execs forthright challenges; adversarial (agency) model with execs lauded or shamed	CEO a dominant personality; Much deferral to his experience, non-Execs able to question; 'embattled' narrative of CEO the main coda	Non-execs robust yet respectful challenge; endemic, framed and legitimated as 'improving patient experience'
Setting I: physical	Large, airy meeting room in Trust HQ Education centre; Non-adversarial 'Horse-shoe' arrangement of tables at the front of the room, space for many observers as required; high quality projection facilities routinely used	Rotating venue, typically cramped, dated and poorly equipped; no consistent seating arrangement; 'audience' very close to board tables	Board room at main site – imposingly furnished (dark wood, large tables); a place 'where important decisions are made'. Separate table for those invited to present to the board – adversarial; calls to mind the layout of an 'inquiry'	Rotating venue, always in well-furnished, low-key 'office' environment. Spacious, with room for a wide range of attendees to observe as required
Setting II: artefacts	Presentations modelled on medical lectures; routinely used to summarise main points of reports in board papers and frame discussion. Successfully limited the scope for alternative challenges	Detailed information presented using software tools; typically 'dry' delivery; used by non-execs to facilitate challenge	Not used other than in 'special' presentations by external speakers – and then not supported by software or projection. Relied on orations from presenters, and challenges made with reference to supporting information in board papers	Presentations routinely used in clinical updates – supported by presentation software and projection facilities
Staging	Highly structured and formal; CEO's report placed early in agenda affording scope to craft an over-arching narrative which reinforced the self-image of the organisation as a high performer even where there were difficulties (e.g. Infection control); Performance data summarised to 1 page of A4 and used to identify 'red' areas for development work – assurance mode	Highly structured and formal; chair steered focus on breach of targets in summary indicators to facilitate robust challenge	CEO dominance of 'matters arising', placed early in the agenda, set the tone. Most of the time spent on these items. The 'CEO show'	Highly structured, yet 'permission to speak'. Opens with a narrative patient story 'to concentrate our minds' – patient experience a guiding principle, invoked routinely. Performance data reported within a 'Quality improvement strategy' section – improvement mode
Performing: infection control	Despite existence of summary A4 'traffic light' indicators showing breach on infection control, CEO used their report to frame perceptions (successful reclassification with commissioners and Monitor) to remove the breach. There was no non-exec challenge.	chair adopts tone of 'disappointment' at data presented on C. diff target breach to demand action by the Nurse Director. No attempt to 'explain away' or contextualise the breach	C. diff targets presented as unobtainable by CEO; Legal challenge threatened to commissioners as part of 'embattled' narrative	Infection control target (reported in QI strategy section) is met but CEO warns against complacency. Data is disaggregated to identify potential 'hot spots' to further drive performance

A dramaturgy of board governance of patient safety

Scripting
While often commenting on information presented to the board, at Arran NEDs were limited in their challenges to executives and avoided overt conflict. In marked contrast the chair and non-executive directors at Skye confidently challenged executives, particularly in relation to poor performance in infection control and capacity issues, demanding that the CEO improve standards. There was clear differentiation in the way that different executives were seen and treated, being either lauded or shamed. The medical director (MD) was widely seen as competent and dependable, and his pathway development work was formally acknowledged:

Chair: Can we please congratulate [Chief Operating Officer name] and [MD name] they're doing a great job.
NED: Yes, the Medical Director is bringing it down to local levels which is great to see ... (Field note extract)

In contrast, the Nurse Director received tougher questioning and her hesitancy was drawn to attention (considered in detail below in the section on 'performance').

At Lewis, board meetings could be summarised as the 'CEO show'; the dominant narrative was of an embattled trust, fighting for local interests – a trust under fire enmeshed in structural, legal and financial disputes. This strongly adversarial framing is typical and exemplified in the CEOs threat to resign in the face of fierce opposition from external opponents:

CEO: It's insulting quite frankly. We're dealing with animals ... I'm willing to resign if this drags on and isn't resolved. (Field note extract)

The CEO's views were rarely challenged internally, with board members supporting his position and accepting his performance as part of the ritual and crafted with humour, emotion, and political point-scoring. The chair had a supportive presence, summarising issues as appropriate.

At Islay the board maintained a clear focus on strategy and service improvement. The CEO projected a calm influence; a moderniser with a similarly oriented executive team who had received quality improvement training which clearly informed board practice. Robust yet respectful challenge was normalised among non-executives, framed and legitimated as 'improving patient experience'. Board dynamics were driven by this central narrative, which granted permission for depersonalised challenge, exemplified in the following field note extract concerning theatre safety, in which improvement activity is explored dispassionately in relation to standardisation and cultural change, rather than personal challenge:

NED: The human factors training is important but has the culture changed? I need to push you that we want to take it forward.
Clinical   We do adhere to the protocols but we constantly want to be individuals as well ...
Lead:
CEO: This is the most challenging area, it should be processed, your personal leadership is needed ... but there needs to be some kind of standardisation.
MD: [name] has been amending the checklist to accommodate different interpretations.... If you go round now, as a result of these changes, you'll see the difference ... The problem was the theatre culture; we need a change of attitude related to infection control. The drive for quality and safety's the most important (Field note extract)

Setting I: physical
Arran board meetings were held within the education centre at Trust HQ in a large room with high-quality presentation facilities. The location reinforced a sense of 'information transmission' (passive) rather than deliberation (active). The room was large, bright and airy, the audience typically consisting of five governors and/or members of the public, ordered into rows of (sparsely populated) chairs facing presentation screens and set back from board members, themselves seated in a 'horseshoe' arrangement of three tables at the front of the room; a non-adversarial setting consistent with a 'common purpose'.

Skye meetings were held at different locations across the trust. With one exception, meeting rooms were cramped, hot, and lacking air circulation. Because of the poor conditions the audience (3–5 governors) tended to split into two groups at opposite sides of the room, very close to the board table. The chair, chief Executive, trust secretary and trust minute-taker sat together, with other seats haphazardly assigned with no consistency across meetings.

Board meetings at Lewis were held at the board room at the main trust site whose décor consisted of dark wood tables and chairs with red leather covers; an imposing environment reflecting civic pride. The seating arrangement was stable across meetings. The chair, chief executive and observers sat together, the business development director and non-executives together on an adjacent table and the nurse and finance director with some spaces for guest speakers and observers. The trust secretary, medical director, and more non-executives sat at an adjacent table. Those invited to present to the board faced an experience akin to an inquiry; waiting in an anteroom for the appointed time on the agenda, invited in when required, positioned on a table in front of the board to face questions, and escorted out once their item concluded.

While the venue for Islay board meetings rotated, all were held in well-furnished, low-key 'office' environments. Rooms were spacious and accommodated observers. Seating was arranged around a large single table on an *ad hoc* basis. Attendees included members of the quality improvement team, and clinical leads who attended to report updates regarding specific clinical reviews.

Setting II: artefacts
Board papers   All sites provided a briefing pack of information ahead of the meeting, consisting of a formal, standardised agenda and appended reports for agenda items in sequence. The format and contents were similar across sites. Two frames of reference underpinned board papers: RAG (red-amber-green) ratings and 'narrative' executive summaries. Board papers presented information in the form of an executive summary of the 'key issues' over the past month and the options for moving forward, and additional quantitative material included line graphs, run charts and bar charts related to performance.

Presentations   At Arran presentations were undertaken by medical staff in response to specific issues highlighted within prior board meetings. The format broadly adhered to conventions associated with academic medical lectures, presenters using available electronic facilities to display detailed presentations, summarising the main points of associated reports appended within the compendium of board papers, and responding to questions from the floor. While affording Non-executive board members the opportunity to raise detailed questions, presenters framed material to anticipate questions and structure the following discussion.

While similar conventions operated at Skye presentations were more informal in tone, lacked vibrancy and afforded Non-executive board members the opportunity to raise questions in relation to detail.

Staging

Formal in operation, the ordering of the agenda at Arran facilitated the crafting of an over-arching narrative by the CEO presenting the organisation as a high performer – even where more detailed reporting suggested potential difficulties.

The detailed 'performance report' delivered by the director of strategy provided a high-level summary and narrative overview of key performance indicator (KPI) data related to activity, efficiency, access, cancer, infection, quality and safety, workforce, finance, and the monitor compliance framework. Performance data were presented for the current month and year to date summarised on a single A4 page, and disaggregated by sub-division (medicine, surgery and cancer, specialist) with additional data in a supporting document. While the structure (KPIs) and form ('traffic-light' RAG indication of performance against targets) of reporting used to inform the board potentially supported the adversarial discharge of public governance in the form of assurance ('conformance'), Non-executives did not use the data to publicly challenge executives at any of the observed board meetings.

The CEO avoided such overt challenges by contextualising shortfalls detailed in the performance report in his preceding 'CEO report', offering an interpretation of figures and outlining on-going work to diagnose and/or address shortfall. We consider this in further detail in the 'performance' section below. The CEO's report was wide-ranging, provided opportunities for clarification and discussion, and consequently took considerable time. The CEO used this composite section, delivered very early in the board meeting, to consider multiple items related to trust activity/performance and their implications, in the light of external policy directives and/or the strategic opportunities they provided.

In contrast to the close executive control above, at Skye the staging was typified by the chair's dominance. His steering of the agenda, and contributions from others, focused principally on the breach of targets (particularly C. difficile (C. diff)) and issues related to coding and validity of statistics, with very limited external horizon scanning or evidence of wider strategy. The chair was active throughout, particularly so in relation to quality and patient safety, evidenced in steering challenges to the nurse director about infection control and the failure to achieve the C. diff target. There was a sense (picked up by an audience member in an aside to researchers) that he dominated the meeting. By controlling the staging and encouraging NED interjections the chair prevented other narratives from unfolding.

Staging at Lewis was shaped by an extensive 'matters arising' section placed immediately after the opening item of 'apologies'. This was by far the longest section and invariably consisted of the following issues considered most important including a major capital investment project; qualified provider procurements; an academic health science network; and commissioner penalties in relation to C. difficile.

In contrast, board meetings at Islay were tightly structured around the agenda. The tone of each meeting was set by an opening 'patient story' narrative, introduced by the chair as 'something to focus our minds'. These narratives, collected by the improvement team, concerned issues such as the fears, anxieties and negative experiences following diagnosis, processes of care and treatment outcomes. They were emotive and used by the chair to legitimate challenge and concern with service improvement; the language of 'patient experience' was available to, and used by, board members to depersonalise challenging questions. Strategic focus on service improvement was supported by the agenda structure, 'service improvement' placed as a standing agenda item immediately after the 'patient story', and led by members of the quality improvement team presenting data and updating progress on strategically important projects including intensive care, community services, falls and infections. The incorporation of indicators for infections into this section is important, as it ties external regulatory requirements to internal strategy in an agenda item specifically oriented to service improvement.

Performance(s): board governance of infection control
Board meetings at Arran were dominated by the CEO and typified by a need to present trust performance in a favourable light, consistent with a 'world-class' reputation. This dominance was not exercised through explicit force of personality, but principally through careful structuring of the agenda and the use of framing in the 'CEO Report' agenda item to shape perceptions of, and thus actions in relation to, items appearing later in the agenda.

As outlined above, the CEO's report drew attention to shortfalls in performance. Notable examples in relation to patient safety included failure to achieve reduction in C. diff targets for three quarters in succession, and a potential breach of A&E waiting time target in the fourth quarter (and thus for the whole year). While both of these topics could have raised vociferous challenges from non-executives, no such challenges were made. Rather, in relation to the former, the CEO announced that commissioners had waived penalties for eight cases, and on this basis he had conferred with the external regulatory body for reclassification as 'green' (healthy) under their governance performance indicator, previously flagged as amber and placing the trust under external scrutiny. This was presented as evidence of over-sensitivity to borderline non-compliance:

CEO: Monitor reports C. diff in A&E is now [six over target] but there are eight cases that we have appealed. These shouldn't have been in the figures in the first place; it should have been identified before coming in (…) we have missed (the target) for three quarters (…) So the problems with A&E combined with C. diff means our governance rating's likely to go down the fourth quarter. It means the organisation hasn't deteriorated but it can give a negative impression to the outside world. (Field note extract)

In the case of the A&E issue, the seriousness of the potential breach was minimised by reference to the ubiquity of such problems ('everyone faces such difficulties'), addressed with reference to current plans to expand A&E provision ('we are already dealing with this'), and attention focused on the role of limited out-of-hours cover by GPs in increasing demand on A&E services ('the problem lies elsewhere').

In both instances, the CEO's report identified poor performance against indicators that could have been addressed as 'breaches', pre-interpreting the data as misleading. That these analyses were convincing is clear from the fact that neither of these issues were picked up by non-executives for further exploration during the subsequent detailed performance report. Given the important work involved in framing these issues the CEO report was typically one of the longer, and on one occasion the longest, agenda item(s) at 46 minutes out of a total of 110 (42% of the total time).

In contrast, board performances at Skye were typified by high levels of NED activity. In relation to breach of a C. diff target, the chair adopted a tone of disappointment at failure to reach the target – presented as a serious issue which needed to be tackled, requiring explanation by the director of nursing. There was no serious attempt to reframe the target breach; the ND is held responsible:

Chair: We've not got continuous quality improvement for C. diff. This has increased from last year which in my opinion is unacceptable … So, is the C-Diff policy in place <name>?

ND: The policy and plan is good, but [she hesitates]

NED: I feel there was a struggle to answer, I'm disappointed with the reaction from the new Nursing Director. (Field note extract)

Detailed discussion followed on the implications for the trust:

NED: What about costs?

FD: Seven over [and] it's a £3.5 million fine, so we need to talk to Commissioners, plus the cost of additional cleaning.

NED: How likely will the surplus be wiped out?

FiD: CCG won't want us bankrupt but there are higher powers than the CCG. (Field note extract)

High levels of challenge were also evident in relation to other performance issues, including a 'red' rating against A&E performance and a lower than anticipated level of emergency admissions.

At Lewis, CEO dominance and use of humour, emotion and politics is exemplified in discussions of a breach of infection control targets. Discussion focused on the financial penalties associated with breach of the target, the trust facing a fine of over £1 million per excess case. Disputes with commissioners ensued and legal proceedings developed, board discussions centred on 'proportionality' and perceived unfair treatment in comparison with regional neighbours:

MD: There's no drive for improvement. [local rival] has had the same target as last year. Why have we been given such a challenging target? [Local rival] isn't in breach of contract even if they miss target! I mean we could use the money and reinvest in community if we are in surplus.... I need a steer if we're not budging on £1.3 million then court mediation is the answer ... It's ridiculous, it's a disincentive to improve, make improvements. We're also going to discuss this with the FT network. The penalties are completely disproportionate....

Non-exec: Yeah, they've got the process wrong here.

Chief   Yes, I know, I've heard [local rival #2] is at <70 more than trust>. We accept
executive: <target> but it's not proportionate. (Field note extract)

The CEO suggested they had no choice but to take commissioners to court as an act of safeguarding local services:

CEO: Someone has to stand up for the NHS and it's going to be <Trust name>. We are going to....

NED: London will be imposing further penalties; I'm pretty sure of that based on my intelligence working with London,

CEO: This isn't about London, this is about the NHS. It's about people delivering the services, people receiving services ... (Field note extract)

While board consideration of infection control at Islay was also framed in relation to external targets, its service improvement orientation was very evident. The MD presented data showing that the trust was meeting its target. This was warmly welcomed by a non-executive who praised the effort, and then quickly considers the interventions required to ensure continuous compliance, prompting a discussion of the educational interventions being made to embed infection control in staff behaviour:

MD: We are under trajectory, we are making good progress. MRSA is an area of anxiety. We had an outbreak on <ward name>, fogging, deep cleaning all as you would expect. A root cause analysis of all cases couldn't find anything. No cause found. It was just patient specific. For E-Coli ... we are trying to distinguish the ones that we can prevent and the ones that are unpreventable.

NED: These are fantastic results to be under the targets but work to be done to assure and provide more details. We need to work within the Divisions with the high turnover of junior doctors in order to educate them about infections; otherwise it's never going to end.

A&E consultant 1:   It's the ownership

Consultant 2:   It's getting permanent staff to communicate with junior doctors and it's also about getting Advanced Nurse Practitioners involved. (Field note extract)

These very different emphases and approaches across sites are summarised in Table 2.

Discussion

Obtaining, processing and interpreting performance information are acknowledged as important aspects of boards' oversight role (Department of Health 2013). While there is limited empirical support internationally that those hospital boards which prioritise the collection and analysis of performance data tend to have improved quality outcomes (Jiang *et al.* 2009), our analysis draws attention to the mediating role played by processing and interpreting performance data and to the performativities at play during deliberation. Consistent with a socio-cultural perspective (Lamont and Waring 2015), performative analysis enables empirically grounded exploration of the refraction of external requirements for patient safety governance through local practices. Specifically, we highlighted the practices involved in realising the potential of patient safety performance indicators (Freeman 2002), and more importantly how the 'warning signals' provided by such data may be muted, deflected or silenced. We consider further the implications of our analysis for recent international empirical research findings, specifically time spent on patient safety; availability of patient safety indicators; and the training required by board members. While cautious of the reification involved in lauding specific interventions as 'solutions' to patient safety problems, we maintain that close analysis of the understandings and conventions in board interactions may be helpful in informing action.

A very high proportion of English NHS hospital Trust boards carry out processes that international research indicates may be associated with higher performance (Jha and Epstein 2013, Mannion *et al.* 2015). All report quality sub-committees (Jha and Epstein 2010) and almost all have explicit objectives related to improving patient safety (Jiang *et al.* 2008, 2009). All of our case study sites sought to provide strategic assurance by establishing organisational structures and processes for reporting safety-related information throughout the organisation and to the board (Botje *et al.* 2014, Jiang *et al.* 2009); making patient safety a strategic priority (Jiang *et al.* 2008); developing and nurturing an 'open and fair culture' (Vaughn *et al.*

2006); and using high level information to ensure compliance with safe practices/standards and external targets (Jha and Epstein 2010). Yet, the degree to which aspirations were fully met was moot, and governance activities remain contingent on board dynamics. Our case study sites exhibited governance behaviours variously related to: agency theory (Chambers and Cornforth 2010), in seeking to measure performance to ensure compliance and hold staff accountable for their actions; stewardship theory (Cornforth and Edwards 1998), in attempting to implement a framework of shared values built on trust; stakeholder theory (Chambers and Cornforth 2010), in managing complex trade-offs between stakeholders, including staff, patients and the public; and resource dependency theory (Zahra and Pearce 1989) in managing internal and external relationships to leverage influence.

Our analysis highlights the role of, and differences in, local processes of organising in relation to board governance of patient safety. Thus while the amount of board time devoted to discussing patient safety has been identified as potentially important (Jha and Epstein 2010), we draw attention to the fact that boards used this time differently. Similarly, while the availability of summary data has been indicated as important (Jiang *et al.* 2008, 2009), and similar levels of performance indicator data relating to infection control were available at each of our case study sites, differences in use were significant and related to the practices legitimated within each setting. At Skye, Arran and Lewis attention focused on data indicating shortfalls – a quality assurance oriented approach. Operationalising the governance of patient safety largely in terms of assurance through retrospective use of performance data to alert the board of poor performance encourages under-reporting and does not indicate how to address deficiencies. Specific responses noted at our sites included challenge and blame by NEDs at Skye; interpretive work by the CEO to forestall challenge at Arran; and framing targets as unrealistic and requiring challenge of regulators at Lewis.

Our results also have implications for the nature of training required by boards. Findings highlighted the challenges board members face in terms of scripting and staging, especially when decisions in these areas often pass unchallenged, unremarked or even unnoticed. A better understanding of these issues may feed into revised training and induction processes for board members. In the USA, a number of states have introduced initiatives in the form of mandatory induction and orientation programmes for board members (Jha and Epstein 2012) and this may also be an area that requires greater attention in the UK. Crucially, while the availability of information may be a necessary precursor for improvement, it is not of itself sufficient. While development of technical 'competencies' in analysis of performance indicators may be helpful, the important role played in setting, scripting and staging in the use and interpretation of information and performance data suggests that a broader curriculum is required directly attending to these issues. While summary reporting of quality indicators is important (Jha and Epstein 2010), local processes of organising that make it possible for non-executive board members to use such information to hold executives to account sensitively are required – most evident at Islay and rather less so elsewhere. Thus the dramaturgical arrangements of boards require attention if they are to become fora for effective debate, challenge and the instigation of action.

Only at Islay did the board seek to provide a strategic focus on quality improvement (to the extent of structuring the board agenda around strategic quality improvement initiatives). This approach seemingly offers a way of managing tensions between assurance and improvement by combining the requirements of external assurance with ongoing quality improvement through development of national and local level datasets, and required additional qualitative information from reports by teams from clinical service areas.

It is important to note that we do not claim privileged status for our own analysis, or suggest that our perspective somehow reflects an underlying 'truth' to which we had special access. We do not claim that the performance indicator data presented at these board meetings showed deficiencies in patient safety that were inappropriately interpreted away. Indeed, the very value of a performative approach is that it traces the way in which words both 'say' and 'do'; to consider meaningful actions that are neither true nor false but create a social reality acted upon by others. Our analysis shows the use of data to create a social reality in relation to infection control rates, which then guided future actions. We would assert however that a set of behaviours/practices that use information to support cycles of improvement activity are required.

Conclusions

Studies of statistical associations between organisational structures and patient safety outcomes are not able to explore the dynamic and messy lived reality of board governance practices related to patient safety (Millar *et al.* 2013). Our analysis of such practices at four Hospital boards indicates the importance of local processes of organising in relation to governance of patient safety. While the availability of summaries of quality indicators to board members is undoubtedly important, so equally are the operation of processes of organising that make it possible for local actors to use such information to make interventions to sensitively hold executives to account with regard to patient safety processes and outcomes. In this regard, our findings indicate the challenges faced by board members in terms of the artefacts at their disposal and the limitations of the scripts and staging associated with board practices. Encouragingly, in drawing attention to practices associated with the enactment of safety and quality they also indicate possibilities and opportunities for enhanced deliberation of information with which to improve the corporate governance of safety and quality, and we encourage additional applications of performativity-based approaches.

Acknowledgements

The authors would like to thank the editor and reviewers for their helpful comments and suggestions in developing this chapter. The research was funded by the National Institute for Health Research (NIHR) Health Services and Delivery Research (HS&DR) programme (grant no. 10/1007/02; project title 'Effective board governance of safe care'; co-applicants R. Mannion, T. Freeman and HTO Davies). The views and opinions expressed therein are those of the authors and do not necessarily reflect those of the HS&DR programme or the Department of Health.

References

Austin, J.L. (1962) *How to Do Things with Words.* Cambridge, MA: Harvard University Press.
Baker, G.R., Denis, J.L., Pomey, M.P. and MacIntosh-Murray, A. (2010) *Effective Governance for Quality and Patient Safety in Canadian Healthcare Organizations: A Report to the Canadian Health Services Research Foundation and the Canadian Patient Safety Institute.* Ottawa: CHSRF/CPSI
Bateson, G. (1972) *Steps to an Ecology of Mind: Collected Essays in Anthropology.* Chicago, IL: University of Chicago Press.
Botje, D., Klazinga, NS, Suñol, R., Groene, O., Pfaff, H., Mannion, R., Depaigne-Loth, A., Arah, OA, Dersarkissian, M. & Wagner, C. (2014) Is having quality as an item on the executive board agenda associated with the implementation of quality management systems in European hospitals: a quantitative analysis, *International Journal of Quality in Health Care*, Suppl 1: 92–9.

Butler, J. (1993) *Bodies that Matter: On the Discursive Limits of 'Sex'*. London: Routledge.

Butler, J. (2010) Performative agency, *Journal of Cultural Economy*, 3, 2, 147–61.

Callon, M. (2007). What Does it Mean to Say that Economics is Performative? In MacKenzie, D., Muniesa, F. and Siu, L. (eds.), *Do Economists Make Markets? On the Performativity of Economics*, Princeton: Princeton University Press, 311–57.

Chambers, N. & Cornforth, C. (2010) The role of corporate governance and boards in organisation performance. In Walshe, K. & Harvey, G. (eds.), *From Knowing to Doing: Connecting Knowledge and Performance in Public Services*, Cambridge: Cambridge University Press, 99–127.

Cornforth, C.J. and Edwards, C. (1998) *Good Governance: Developing Effective Board-Management Relations in Public and Voluntary Organisations*. London: CIMA Publications.

Currie, G., Humphreys, M., Waring, J. & Rowley, E. (2009) Narratives of professional regulation and patient safety: the case of medical devices in anaesthetics, *Health, Risk and Society*, 11, 117–35.

Czarniawska, B. and Sevon, G. (1996) Introduction. In Czarniawska, B. and Sevon, G. (eds.), *Translating Organizational Change*, Berlin: de Gruyter.

Department of Health (2000) *An Organisation with a Memory*. London: Stationery Office.

Department of Health (2013) *A Promise to Learn – a Commitment to Act: Improving the Safety of Patients in England*. London: Stationery Office.

Diedrich, A., Walter, L. and Czarniawska, B. (2011) Boundary stories: constructing the validation centre in west Sweden, *Scandinavian Journal of Public Administration*, 15, 1, 3–20.

Dr. Foster (2011) *The Good Hospital Guide*. London: Dr. Foster Intelligence.

Feldman, M. and Pentland, B. (2003) Reconceptualizing organizational routines as a source of flexibility and change, *Administrative Science Quarterly*, 48, 1, 94–118.

Francis, R. (2013) *The Mid Staffordshire NHS Foundation Trust Public Inquiry*. London: Stationery Office.

Freeman, T. (2002) Using performance indicators to improve health care quality in the public sector: a review of the literature, *Health Services Management Research*, 15, 2, 126–37.

Freeman, T. and Peck, E. (2007) Preforming governance: a partnership board dramaturgy, *Public Administration*, 85, 4, 907–29.

Freeman, T. and Peck, E. (2010) Culture made flesh: discourse, performativity and materiality. In Braithwaite, J., Hyde, P. and Pope, C. (eds.), *Culture and Climate in Health Care Organizations*, Basingstoke: Palgrave Macmillan.

Goffman, E. (1959) *The Presentation of Self in Everyday Life*. New York: Doubleday.

Goffman, E. (1974) *Frame analysis: An essay on the organization of experience*, Boston: Northeastern University Press.

Hajer, M. (2005) Setting the stage: a dramaturgy of policy deliberation, *Administration and Society*, 36, 6, 624–47.

Hajer, M. and Versteeg, W. (2005) Performing governance through networks, *European Political Science*, 4, 3, 340–7.

Institute of Medicine (1999) *To Err Is Human: Building a Safer Health System*. Washington, DC: National Academy Press.

Jha, A.K. and Epstein, A.M. (2010) Hospital governance and the quality of care, *Health Affairs*, 29, 1, 182–7.

Jha A.K. and Epstein, A.M. (2012) Governance around Quality of Care at Hospitals That Disproportionately Care for Black Patients, *Journal of General Internal Medicine*, 27, 3, 297–303.

Jha, A.K. and Epstein, A.M. (2013) A survey of board chairs in English hospitals shows greater attention to quality of care than among their US counterparts, *Health Affairs*, 32, 4, 677–85.

Jiang, H.J., Lockee, C., Bass, K. and Fraser, I. (2009) Board oversight of quality: any differences in process of care and mortality?, *Journal of Healthcare Management*, 54, 1, 15–30.

Jiang, H.J., Lockee, C., Bass, K. and Fraser, I. (2011) Enhancing board oversight on quality of hospital care: an agency theory perspective, *Health Care Management Review*, 37, 2, 44–53.

Lamont, T. and Waring, J. (2015) Safety lessons: shifting paradigms and new directions for patient safety research, *Journal of Health Services Research and Policy*, 20, 1S, 1–8.

Latour, B. (1986) The powers of association. In Law, J. (ed.), *Power Action and Belief*, London: Routledge and Keegan Paul.

Latour, B. (1987) *Science in Action: How to Follow Scientists and Engineers through Society.* Cambridge, MA: Harvard University Press.

Law, J. and Singleton, V. (2000) Performing technology's stories: on social constructivism, performance and performativity, *Technology and Culture*, 41, 4, 765–75.

Lyotard, J. (1979) *The Postmodern Condition: A Report on Knowledge.* Manchester: Manchester University Press.

Macrae, C. (2014) *Close Calls.* London: Palgrave Macmillan.

Mannion, R., Davies, H.T.O., Freeman, T., Millar, R., Jacobs, R. & Kasteridis, P. (2015) Overseeing oversight: governance of quality and safety by hospital boards in the English NHS, *Journal of Health Services Research and Policy*, 20, 1S, 9–16.

Millar, R., Mannion, R., Freeman, T. and Davies, H.T.O. (2013) Hospital board oversight of patient safety: a narrative review and synthesis of relevant empirical research, *Milbank Quarterly*, 91, 4, 738–70.

Nelson, E.C., Godfrey, M.M., Batalden, P.B., Berry, S.A., Bothe, A.E. Jr., McKinley, K.E., Melin, C.N., Muething, S.E., Moore, L.G., Wasson, J.H. and Nolan, T.W. (2008) Clinical microsystems, part 1. The building blocks of health systems, *Joint Commission Journal Quality and Patient Safety*, 34, 7, 367–78.

NHS Leadership Academy (2013) The Healthy NHS board: Principles for good governance, London: NHS Leadership Academy. Available at http://www.leadershipacademy.nhs.uk/wp-content/uploads/2013/06/NHSLeadership-HealthyNHSboard-2013.pdf. Last accessed 24th July 2015.

Nicolini, D., Waring, J. and Mengis, J. (2011) Policy and practice in the use of root cause analysis to investigate clinical adverse events: Mind the gap, *Social Science and Medicine*, 73, 2, 217–25.

Orlikowski, W.J. and Scott, S. (2008) Sociomateriality: challenging the separation of technology, work and organization, *The Academy of Management Annals*, 2, 1, 433–74.

Ramsay, A., Magnusson, C. and Fulop, N. (2010) The relationship between external and local governance systems: the case of health care associated infections and medication errors in one NHS trust, *Quality & Safety in Health Care*, 19, 6, 1–8.

Rowley, E. and Waring, J. (2011) *A socio-cultural perspective on patient safety*, Farnham: Ashgate.

Sheldon, T.A., Cullum, N., Dawson, D., Lankshear, A., Lowson, K., Watt, I., West, P., Wright, D. & Wright, J. (2004) What's the evidence that NICE guidance has been implemented? Results from a national evaluation using time series analysis, audit of patients' notes, and interviews, *British Medical Journal*, 329, 7473, 999–1006.

Stake, R.E. (1995) *The Art of Case Study Research.* Thousand Oaks, CA: Sage.

Vaughn, T., Koepke, M., Kroch, E., Lehrman, W., Sinha, S. and Levey, S. (2006) Engagement of leadership in quality improvement initiatives: Executive quality improvement surveys, *Journal of Patient Safety*, 2, 1, 2–9.

Waring, J. (2007) Adaptive regulation or governmentality: patient safety and the changing regulation of medicine, *Sociology of Health & Illness*, 29, 2, 163–79.

Waring, J., Rowley, E., Dingwall, R., Palmer, C. and Murcott, T. (2010) A narrative review of the UK Patient Safety Research Portfolio, *Journal of Health Services Research and Policy*, 15, 1, 26–32.

Zahra, S. and Pearce, J. (1989) Boards of directors and corporate financial performance: a review and integrative model, *Journal of Management*, 15, 2, 291–334.

5

The social practice of rescue: the safety implications of acute illness trajectories and patient categorisation in medical and maternity settings

Nicola Mackintosh and Jane Sandall

Introduction

In line with the modern ordering of social phenomena (Bayatrizi 2008: 51), the acutely ill patient has become 'an object of interest, inquiry, demystification, quantification, surveillance and regulation'. In this chapter we seek to extend the body of literature on patient eligibility, categorisation and disposal (that is, the next stage of intervention, treatment or transfer) beyond the emergency department to maternity and the general medical ward. We explore the social practice of rescue, in particular the sociocultural influences that guide the categorisation and ordering of acutely ill patients in these different hospital settings. The chapter's novelty lies in its consideration of meso-level and micro-level ordering practices in conjunction with patients' acute illness trajectories. Our investigation adds to the sociological literature on both categorisation and illness trajectories. It also shifts conceptualisations of managing acute illness beyond bounded individual and team features and instrumental notions of safety solutions, to acknowledge in addition links with wider socio-political influences, including the management of institutional risk.

A focus on rescue in the context of acute illness

Providing an effective safety net for patients in general hospital wards involves the surveillance and timely or appropriate management of patients whose conditions may vary from stable to acutely unwell. The onset of critical illness appears to be often predictable (Schein *et al.* 1990). More effective rescue at an earlier stage is likely to lead to both health and economic gains by reducing cardiac arrests, intensive care unit (ICU) admissions and mortality rates (Buist *et al.* 1999, Hodgetts *et al.* 2002). This includes the timely management of severe maternal morbidity (for example, sepsis, post-partum haemorrhage and pre-eclampsia). In this chapter we focus on critical illness in the high stake settings of general medicine and maternity. Both specialties are undergoing rapid innovation in service delivery, and are characterised by changes in patients' characteristics, workforce roles and responsibilities and shifting interfaces with other services (for example, primary care, emergency departments and critical care).

Ward profiles in acute care have become more complex, resulting in increased patient acuity and a higher workload as a result of greater take-up of healthcare technology and the

The Sociology of Healthcare Safety and Quality, First Edition. Edited by Davina Allen, Jeffrey Braithwaite, Jane Sandall and Justin Waring. Chapters © 2016 The Authors. Book Compilation © 2016 Foundation for the Sociology of Health & Illness/Blackwell Publishing Ltd.

need to care for an ageing population with multiple comorbidities (Bion and Heffner 2004). In this environment, opportunities for rescue are often missed. There is widespread evidence of ward staff's failure to recognise warning signs of deterioration and difficulties in interpreting and instituting appropriate clinical management once concerns have been identified (National Confidential Enquiry into Patient Outcome and Death [NCEPOD] 2005, National Patient Safety Agency 2007).

Maternity services are also under strain, partly as a consequence of an increasing birth rate, and a population of mothers that is generally older than they used to be, with some groups experiencing more comorbidities (National Audit Office 2013, Royal College of Midwives 2013). The volume of births to women born outside the UK has also risen; these mothers often have more complicated pregnancies, have more serious underlying medical conditions or may be in poorer general health than women born in the UK (Centre for Maternal and Child Enquiries [CMACE] 2011). While for the most part, pregnancy and birth are normal physiological processes, emergencies can develop rapidly and unexpectedly. Delayed detection of severe illness in women before, during and after childbirth can lead to poor outcomes for women and their babies (CMACE 2011).

Current risk management strategies in maternity and acute care settings include a plethora of safety systems and tool kits, such as vital sign charts and care protocols to standardise escalation pathways (King's Fund 2012, National Institute of Health and Clinical Excellence [NICE] 2007), track and trigger tools and decision aids to shape the interpretation of clinical deterioration and appropriate intervention (CMACE 2011, NICE 2007); communication protocols to provide junior staff with the mandate to ask for help (King's Fund 2012, NICE 2007); individual and team training to improve ward staff skills in recognition and response (Smith *et al.* 2002) and outreach or medical emergency teams to provide access to specialist support (Winters *et al.* 2013). Despite these, management of acute illness remains problematic (CMACE 2011, NCEPOD 2012).

We suggest that widening the analytical lens beyond individual and team processes and technical safety solutions may enhance our understanding of why management of the acutely ill represents such a 'wicked problem'. Wicked problems are those that are difficult or impossible to solve on account of their contradictory nature and associated interdependencies, which mean that solving one aspect may lead to fresh problems (Rittel and Weber 1973). Drawing on sociological concepts of patient trajectories and categorisation enables us to situate rescue practice in the wider social practice of hospital care, and thereby usefully examine associated context, congruencies, complexities and tensions.

Managing patients' trajectories in hospital settings

Strauss *et al.*'s (1985) notion of the patient trajectory offers a useful theoretical resource for the study of rescue, since it encompasses not only the unfolding pathology of the patient condition but also the organisational work undertaken to accomplish that trajectory, and its consequences for the relationships between those involved. They suggest that technological specialisation and the complex bureaucracy of healthcare have resulted in fragmentation of care processes. They identify two characteristic features to healthcare work. Firstly, unexpected contingencies arise from both patients' disease processes and a whole range of organisational and technological sources. Secondly, patients react to and affect healthcare work. These combined features create the potential for trajectories of care to be complex and highly problematic.

Strauss *et al.* (1997) observe that the extent to which various dangers and risks associated with the trajectory phases can be mapped out determines the coordination of the total arc of work, including the bundles of implicated tasks. They distinguish between trajectories where an illness is well understood, and which are amenable to control by standardised policies, and highly problematic trajectories that involve attendant uncertainties:

> These uncertainties greatly increase the probability and even cumulative impact of certain kinds of mistakes stemming from the tasks themselves, from possible consequences of doing the tasks and even from the organisation of error work itself, which can lead to unanticipated new mistakes (Strauss *et al.* 1997: 243).

Various authors have usefully drawn on Strauss' writings to progress understanding of the linkages between individual trajectories of care and broader health and social care systems (Allen *et al.* 2004, Mesman 2008). We extend the use of Strauss *et al.*'s work to include the hospital ward setting (including the maternity unit), and to situate the coordination of patient trajectories of clinical deterioration with other types of clinical work, ward cultures and temporal-spatial influences.

Categorisation and ordering practices

The sociological literature on ordering practices offers an additional framework to examine sense-making regarding acutely ill patients. Roth (2005) notes that while ordering practices are ordinarily unproblematic and invisible, 'the concrete world and the processes of differentiation are always situated, local, and saturated with contingencies' (Roth 2005: 584). Roth suggests that there are 'few empirical studies of the real-time production, use and impact of classification in everyday work praxis' (2005: 15). Bowker and Star (1999) agree: 'what is missing is a sense of the landscape of [classification] work as experienced by those within it' (p. 65). In this chapter we attempt to address this gap by articulating the dynamics of the landscape of acute illness in medical and maternity settings.

Calculations around prognosis and acuity differ inter-professionally; variance depends to some extent on the different criteria used (Degner and Beaton 1987). Provider rationing on the basis of the candidacy, or eligibility (Dixon-Woods *et al.* 2006) of patients who are considered more or less worthy of care determines the way that particular patients gain access to services (Nugus and Braithwaite 2010). Clinical, social and organisational categorisation work occurs at the point of initial access to hospital care (Dingwall and Murray 1983, Dodier and Camus 1998, Hughes 1980, Jeffery 1979, Vassy 2001). Our interest extends this lens to legitimacy work that takes place in the acute hospital structure. Using this literature in conjunction with theories on patient trajectories enables us to explore meso-level and micro-level distinction practices separating acute illness from other categories, and the consequences of this and other sociocultural factors for patients' trajectories.

The research project

Within the context of a national policy imperative on the poor management of deterioration in clinical practice, this research was part of a larger programme of National Institute for Health Research (NIHR)-funded work exploring how services are organised to improve patients' journeys through and across care systems. This study aimed to explore how the deterioration and escalation of care are understood in the workplace, and the intended and unintended consequences of safety strategies and tools introduced to facilitate management of acutely ill patients. The study design involved an ethnographic approach over a 2-year period (2009–2010) and was organised into two phases. Data were collected in the medical directorates (> 150 hours of observations, January to December 2009), and then in maternity services (> 120 hours of observations, February to August 2010). Findings on the role of safety systems in medicine (Mackintosh et al. 2011) and maternity (Mackintosh et al. 2013) have been reported. Findings from patients' (30) and relatives' (11) perceptions about their role in contributing to the escalation of care have also been reported (Rainey et al. 2015, Rance et al. 2013). This chapter focuses on the social structuring practices that shape patients' trajectories and draws on staff interviews, observation and documentary data from both maternity and medicine. The analysis of the variation in findings between the two care settings provides insights into relationships between meso-level and micro-level systems.

The ethnographic approach to the study of medical work offered an effective means of uncovering how rescue is accomplished, and the relationships between this work and other structural factors. Ethnographies of work practices reveal 'the unacknowledged, the hidden, the insider knowledge, the unwritten but pervasive rules governing jobs' (Smith 2007: 222). The research was based across two urban inner city hospital trusts. The pseudonyms, Eastward and Westward, maintain the anonymity of the sites. Each Trust's medical directorate consisted of ten wards, altogether admitting 15,000–20,000 patients per year. Each had a maternity service providing care for around 6000 women annually. Eastward had an obstetric unit (mixed high and low risk care environment) while Westward had both an alongside midwifery unit (providing care for women classed as low risk) and an obstetric unit (a predominantly high risk environment). Both trusts provided services for home birth and cared for women who were transferred in from home. Table 1 details structural aspects of the sites. Both organisations were similar in terms of location, population served, admission rates and ward settings.

After ethical and research governance approval was obtained (08/H0808/178), data were collected by the first author (who has a critical care nursing and social science background) in the medical directorates, and by the first author and two additional researchers (one with a midwifery and one with a sociology background) in maternity services. While the selection of a particular field is directed by a theoretical interest in a specific problem, the significance of the many events contextualising the problem can never be determined a priori. Rather than focusing solely on emergency episodes when patients became acutely unwell, we learned about the everyday reality and routines of each area and collected data on space, actors, activities and objects, as well as events and time goals (Robson 1993).

Observation of ward or unit activity and medical work enabled an additional opportunistic focus on events and interactions as they arose. In addition to the unstructured observation of ward and unit work, we shadowed a cross-section of medical staff to gain insight into their routine working day as well as their on-call episodes (Table 2). Recruitment was done by e-mail as well as face to face invitations (via meetings and during fieldwork on the wards). Fieldwork included the observation of management-level meetings about the care of acutely ill patients. Jottings or headnotes were audio-recorded immediately after the conclusion of each day's observations (Emerson et al. 1995) and transcribed.

Interpretations of practice were followed up during in-depth interviews with a range of staff, to test out assumptions and clarify contradictory understandings. Staff members were recruited for interview by a mixture of e-mail and face to face contact. The interviews were conducted in private spaces (offices, meeting rooms and coffee rooms) and lasted between 20 and 70 minutes. Interviewees were purposively selected for their theoretical

Table 1   *Structural features of the two research sites*

Contextual features	Westward	Eastward
Hospital descriptor	UK acute teaching hospital	UK acute teaching hospital
Location	Inner city	Inner city
Demographics	Mobile population, high ethnic diversity	Mobile population, high ethnic diversity
General medical service	15,000–20,000 patients admitted per year	15,000–20,000 patients admitted per year
	10 general medical wards	10 general medical wards
Study ward/beds	General medicine with respiratory specialty/30 beds	General medicine with diabetes specialty/28 beds
Safety systems/tools in use across medical service	Track and trigger tool[1] Critical care outreach team[2]	Track and trigger tool
Maternity service	> 6500 births per year	5500 births per year.
	Obstetric unit, alongside midwifery unit, antenatal/postnatal ward, antenatal day unit	Obstetric unit, antenatal/postnatal ward, maternal assessment unit
Study unit(s)	Obstetric unit alongside midwifery unit	Obstetric unit
Safety systems/tools in use across maternity services	Partogram[3] Track and trigger tool Critical care outreach team	Partogram Track and trigger tool

[1] A set of rules to distinguish when vital signs become of concern and appropriate trigger actions that need to be taken as a result.
[2] A team set up to facilitate management of acutely ill patients on the ward.
[3] A chart to plot the progress of labour to allow for early detection of problems with both mother and baby.

representativeness, in terms of the categories, substructures and networks of the social organisation (Johnson 1990).

All transcripts of observations, interviews, minutes of meetings, and documentary data were imported into N-Vivo version 8. This facilitated content and thematic analysis. The analysis aimed to preserve particular patients' rescue trajectories, including their care provision and interactions, over periods of fieldwork. We drew on the framework approach, which involves a series of interconnected stages that enable the researcher to move back and forth across the data until a coherent account emerges (Ritchie and Lewis 2003). This involved making sense of the core concepts, which had emerged from the refined categories and final themes, the clinical literature and the theoretical sociological perspectives.

Glaser (1998) recommends three codes of increasingly abstract categorisation: substantive, theoretical and core. Five substantive codes were generated: routine work; identification of a problem; asking for help; responding and structural influences. We developed four theoretical codes: enactment of safety work; division of labour; boundary work and socio-technical systems. Rescue work formed the core code. The findings reported in this chapter draw from the structural influences code and link to all four of the theoretical codes. We consider the clinical presentation, categorisation and care of acutely ill patients, and how these relate to wider institutional sociocultural and political influences. These relationships inform comparisons between settings and enable an analysis of the work involved in managing linked processes such as efficiency, responsiveness, effectiveness and safety.

Table 2 *Data collection*

| | Westward | | Eastward | |
	Medical	Maternity	Medical	Maternity
Observations	10 ward shifts, 4 shifts shadowing medical staff, 8 acutely ill patient in hospital committee meetings	4 alongside midwifery unit shifts, 6 obstetric unit shifts, 11 risk meetings	8 ward shifts, 4 shifts shadowing medical staff, 1 shift with outreach team, 10 acutely ill patient in hospital committee meetings	11 obstetric unit shifts 5 risk meetings
Interviews	HCAs: 2 Ward nurses: 3 Outreach nurses: 2 Doctors: 5 Managers: 2 Total: 14	Midwives: 8 Obstetricians: 7 Anaesthetist: 2 Neonatologist: 0 Managers: 6 Total: 23	HCAs: 2 Nurses: 4 Physio: 1 Doctors: 9 Managers: 5 Total: 21	Midwives: 9 Obstetricians: 4 Anaesthetist: 1 Neonatologist: 1 Managers: 6 Total: 21
Documentary review	Ward protocols, audits, minutes of acutely ill patient in hospital committee meetings, ICU admission audits	Ward protocols, audits, minutes of risk meetings	Ward protocols, audits, minutes of acutely ill patient in hospital committee meetings, ICU admission audits 7 months data from intelligent assessment technology	Ward protocols, audits, minutes of risk meetings

HCA, healthcare assistant

Findings

The rescue imperative in the context of maternity and medical care
Across the two care settings, the nature of the clinical emergency and its demands for immediate medical attention emerged as a core organising frame. The rescue imperative underpinned the logic of acute hospital care. The concept of the trajectory (Strauss *et al.* 1985) was important for setting timelines and structuring care in relation to sickness (and death) and birth (De Vries 1981). Both organisations had invested in systems and processes designed to facilitate intervention in the time period preceding the patient's collapse, potentially halting and reversing the trajectory of clinical deterioration and imposing order on the associated unpredictability and crisis. Rescue provided a social and ideological mandate for practice (Chapple 2010). The accomplishment of effective and timely management of clinical deterioration demonstrated the essential business of acute and maternity care delivery, as this consultant physician says:

> We observe patients for signs of deterioration. This is the most basic aspect of hospital care. Here it's done reasonably well, at a level where if you were running a dry cleaning operation if it was much worse you'd be out of business because you'd lose so many suits. (Westward, Physician, 11)[1]

In maternity, the rationality and moral worth of urgent rescue work was particularly evident. While acute events were relatively infrequent on the medical wards, on the obstetric units the management of clinical crises was normalised as part of 'what we do round here'. Discourse on the units frequently involved midwives and doctors recounting atrocity stories (Dingwall 1977) as a means of recognising the accomplishment of heroic rescue work:

> At half past ten the emergency buzzer went off in room 5 so the coordinator and medical staff who were in the office ran to the room. Five, ten minutes later the coordinator came back saying it was a cord prolapse, minutes later the woman was transferred to theatre with one of the doctors astride her, holding the cord up.[2] Once the coordinator had checked all the staff were present in theatre she returned and very quickly the office was quiet again and the rest of the unit appeared to carry on as normal. (Westward, FN7)

The midwives are chatting about the TV programme, 'One Born Every Minute', saying how lovely and cosy that environment was, how it didn't reflect practice 'here'. One midwife recounts an episode showing an emergency transfer of a woman in labour to theatre. She says scornfully 'we would have done it much faster, we would have had her in theatre in seconds, not like the slow process that we saw on telly'. The other two murmur their agreement (Eastward, FN5).

While rescue served as an organising principle across all settings, the enactment of local rescue processes reflected variance in patient groups, sociocultural norms and trajectories of clinical deterioration. An important feature in maternity was the view that the 'women aren't sick, these are women who are young, they are healthy' (Westward, Midwife, 15). Difficulties distinguishing changes associated with normal pregnancy from the signs of acute illness made the recognition of deterioration a complex process: 'Women are incredibly resilient, and can deal with enormous blood loss' (Westward, Anaesthetist, 11). By the time that a woman started to show signs of physiological compromise, the underlying problem was often fairly well advanced, necessitating prompt action to avert avoidable harm for the woman or her child.

In medicine, the pattern of deterioration in physiological observations was reported to provide more of a window of opportunity for detection and intervention than in maternity. Patients could show signs of clinical deterioration for hours or even days as their acute illness developed. The logic of rescue in the acute care setting was linked to the alignment of symptoms and pathology, and the ability to halt and potentially reverse clinical deterioration. As a physician noted:

> We are trying to improve the care of people that are getting sicker in the Trust, by identifying them and identifying pathways by which their condition might be improved. (Westward, Physician, 16)

Ensuring safety, quality and efficiency

Across both settings, a discourse of prediction, control and avoidance of the accidental (Green 2003) provided a frame of reference for managing acute illness. Adverse outcomes such as cardiac arrest, a patient's unexpected admission to intensive care and an unexpected death in hospital represented the mismanagement of illness trajectories. Risk-management techniques had been introduced as a means to engender the public's confidence in the hospital institutions. Problems with rescue, like other patient safety problems, were constructed as amenable to methodological and technical improvement (Jensen 2008):

> It was shameful what went on here [in the past] because awful things happened to patients and there was no systematic quality control or control of process or whatever, it was just, well, night follows day and these things happen. Too often the patients would be allowed to deteriorate and either die or get serious complications or whatever, you know, because of failure of effective recognition and response. [We've recognised] that it's important to quality control management of acutely ill patients. (Westward, Manager, 11)

> We want good outcomes for mothers and babies, therefore it follows when something goes wrong, there should be reasons that can be understood and processes put in place to try and reduce the chances of those things happening in future. (Eastward, Obstetrician, 1)

Track and trigger tools had been introduced to both medical and maternity settings to enable the detection of clinical deterioration. Track and trigger systems are simple algorithms detailing a plan of action based on vital sign measurements. Points are allotted to particular vital sign measurements on the basis of physiological derangement from a predetermined range, generating an 'early warning score'. These systems help shape constructs of deterioration and the point of intervention, and provide legitimacy for calling for help (Mackintosh and Sandall 2010, Mackintosh *et al.* 2014). Escalation pathways had been put in place to ensure that acutely ill patients had access to appropriate critical care services.

In maternity, the added value of the track and trigger system in controlling for risk and 'problematic' trajectories was limited, given there was little prior warning of the event for a number of obstetric complications. Individual midwives and obstetricians were able to resist using the system routinely in the postnatal period on account of concerns that it medicalised normal childbirth trajectories. The potential gain in detecting morbidity early was also perceived to be small when offset against the increase in workload involved in managing follow-up vital sign recordings and false positive referrals.

However, the unpredictability of maternity collapse and the high social worth of women (and their babies) reinforced a need for management and organisational control of rescue practice (Green and Armstrong 1993, Walsh 2006). As Timmermans (1999) noted in his study of resuscitation efforts, value judgements about the patient's age, quality of life and perceived seriousness of the illness render these variables social. Managing trajectories in this setting involved being prepared for a crisis and having the resource to respond quickly to changes at organisational level (unit capacity). Ensuring flow through the system to ensure access to obstetric resource for crisis management was essential for efficiency and effectiveness:

> We have got two patients and our patients aren't patients, they're well and start off entirely normal and then they have life-threatening problems which are unexpected disasters every time. This is not a geriatric ward … Care of these cases is always highly emotional. (Westward, Obstetrician, 1)

Accounting for risks was an important part of securing trust in the maternity service. All obstetric emergencies such as maternal haemorrhage, maternal or infant admission to intensive care, maternal or neonatal infection, stillbirth and maternal death were classed as clinical incidents and investigated:

> Maternity is streets ahead of every other directorate in the Trust [with regards to risk management], because we have so many risks, but there's a much more transparent approach, so if an incident occurs you're likely to get three risk reports rather than nothing. (Westward, Manager, 13)

The risks posed by the poor detection of and response to acute illness were substantial in terms of poor health outcomes for mother and baby, and litigation costs incurred for remedial care and compensation:

> Everybody thinks that if they get pregnant they're going to have a perfect pregnancy and delivery and a perfect baby, and if it goes wrong somebody must be to blame. (Eastward, Obstetrician, 17)

Within the medical ward setting, managing risks and trajectories presented a different set of issues. As one consultant physician explained, 'we have many deaths and many people that are old, frail and sick and probably going to die in the next year' (Eastward, Physician 16). Audit data provided a window to enable managers and clinical leads to distinguish between patients' trajectories and categorise those that were problematic. Certain trajectories were less amenable to control, which had implications for the scope of quality improvement of associated rescue processes. For example, head and neck cancer was associated with sudden catastrophic haemorrhage and coronary events were associated with sudden collapse which limited the opportunity for improving detection and response behaviour:

> Our ultimate goal is that there will be no cardiac arrests in ward areas … With straightforward medical patients there are usually markers [of deterioration] that are present. When we speak to cardiac teams then it's not quite so easy to predict, in the last month the two cardiac areas had the vast majority of the arrests in ward areas. I think that's to do with cardiac physiology. And the other ones that we find have quite a few

arrests are head and neck cancer where the patients haemorrhage. So I've met with the nurse specialist for those patients and she's looking if there's anything that could be done. (Westward, Manager, 10)

While the default position in medical wards was to resuscitate and rescue unless a written mandate specified otherwise, something much closer to an efficacy model was evident in practice, with its emphasis on the appropriateness of resuscitation and the escalation of care orders:

Five of us are at the acutely ill patients' meeting, including a physician (the chair), a palliative care consultant, a clinical governance lead and a critical care nurse. The chair discusses the potential for the Trust to develop three care pathways for all hospital patients: (a) those for active resuscitation (b) those who need resuscitation but ITU [therapy intensive unit] admission may not be in their best interest and (c) those who need palliative care and are not for resuscitation or escalation of care. (Eastward, Field notes 8)

Quality and efficiency frames of reference (Hillman *et al.* 2013) were used to rationalise these distinction practices on the grounds of avoidance of the distress associated with 'misplaced rescue'. At both trusts a number of incident and audit reports of poor decision-making around end of life care and cases of inappropriate resuscitation had contributed to a growing pressure for a change to the way that acute care was provided. At Eastward there was an additional pressure to conserve critical care resources, which were limited in comparison to those at neighbouring trusts:

[This] organisation has limited critical care capacity and has to make prioritisation decisions … Certain patient groups have a relatively high mortality when admitted to a critical care setting namely, patients in chronic renal failure, patients with HIV infection, patients with haematological malignancy, and any patient over 80 years of age. Such patients are at high risk of 'futile' critical care admission … Any patient [with these conditions] or over 80 years of age should automatically trigger a case conference within 48 hours between the admitting consultant and the duty critical care consultant. The case conference should also establish in writing a comprehensive treatment plan to include decisions around escalation and resuscitation. (Excerpt from Eastward critical care policy document, unpublished, 2007)

Selective access to critical care was legitimised to prevent the burden of mortality being shifted from the ward to the intensive care unit, thus diverting resources that could be used for other patients more likely to benefit from this specialist service.

Local systems of categorisation in rescue presented a simplistic picture of clinical work, creating notions of transparency (Tsoukas 1997). Certain additional risks associated with these processes largely escaped organisational attention. We turn first to the hidden problem of managing the deteriorating conditions of elderly patients with complex conditions in medical wards, and secondly, boundary distinctions between maternity rescue resources.

The acutely ill 'crocks' in medical wards

Crocks (Becker 1993) are those patients who have a number of complaints but no discernible pathology and puzzles to solve. Modern healthcare is poorly designed to meet the needs of people with many things wrong at once; these patients are constructed as inappropriate for the system (Rockwood and Hubbard 2004). The inbuilt algorithms for the track and trigger systems used in acute care were designed for an average patient on a hospital ward (Suokas 2010). A number of acutely ill patients on the medical wards presented with more than one chronic condition compounding their acute illness (Tadd *et al.* 2011). Baseline readings for vital signs for elderly patients with complex, long-term conditions often lay outside the normal range or lay close to the thresholds set for the escalation of care. Patients with chronic respiratory disease often triggered a false positive alert even when their condition was stable. The trigger system was less able to discriminate between this stable state and when patients' condition was deteriorating:

> With chronic obstructive pulmonary disease patients … I think sometimes a deterioration in their condition is a lot harder to pick up on, because they've already got low saturations, they've already got high respiratory rates. Sometimes it takes a lot longer for the score to pick up a problem. Whereas someone young who comes in with tuberculosis you pick it up quite quickly because there's nothing else wrong with them, so there's no reason for them to be like that. (Westward, Nurse, 3)

Two types of additional risk for these patients were introduced by the systems. Firstly, there was greater need for nurses to use clinical judgement in assessing the significance of the risk scores and alerts in the light of the patient's specific condition. This was difficult at times, given that the track and trigger systems were designed to provide jurisdictional control over a craftsman-type model of practice (Harrison and Smith 2004). Secondly, a risk associated with persistent over-triggering was the normalisation of high scores. A woman who had a cardiac arrest on one of the wards died later in intensive care after scoring highly for a number of days due to a raised temperature. A history of mental health problems had complicated the presentation of her illness. Over time, the team collectively became conditioned to the patient's raised score:

> We had a mental health patient who was transferred from a psychiatric ward to us with a pyrexia of unknown origin, her temperature was high, had always been high, she'd always been tachycardic [a high heartbeat rate], she'd always had low blood pressure, so when you looked at her pattern it was like normal … well, normal for her, you know. Although it's been the norm, every time I did [the observations] I let somebody know that this is what [the chart] says … The doctor came and reviewed the patient again, but just said to continue with the current plan. (Eastward, Nurse, 4)

Within the medical directorate, the wards were categorised according to particular medical specialties that aligned with these organs, such as cardiology and respiratory, in addition to specialised service wards such as health and ageing, and rehabilitation wards. Patients with more than one condition (as in the example of the mental health patient) were disadvantaged by this categorisation process. These patients often fell through the gaps of the bureaucratic structure of the hospital and escaped timely attention. They became lost between specialisms with no one taking an overview of the person as a whole (Tadd *et al.* 2011):

> When a patient's condition is very complex, lots of teams are involved but often nobody's really taken ownership. The patient can end up being slightly in limbo, with lots of opinions, but no action. Particularly if there is some degree of disagreement between specialties, the end result is that nobody does anything, there's a bit of a waiting game, and the patient continues to deteriorate. (Eastward, Physician, 15)

Because of elderly patients' multiple conditions, their medical teams frequently required specialist advice from other teams (such as neurology or cardiology). Specialist teams were observed to protect the boundaries of their practice. Acceptance of a referral was contingent on evidence of sufficient diagnostic tests and the presence of new, 'interesting' clinical signs and symptoms. Dodier and Camus (1998) observed that interesting cases are those 'that are difficult to solve, but where there is hope of clarification, which excludes rather poorly differentiated conditions such as alterations in the general state of elderly people' (p. 16). The safety and quality of care was compromised for these crocks (Becker 1993):

> On the ward round we see Fred who is an elderly man who collapsed at home. His medical team have sought advice from the neurology team as they are unsure if his collapse is cardiac or neurological in origin. The neurology team have declined to review Fred this admission as they have already seen him recently in the outpatient clinic. (Westward, Field notes 11)

Underpinning risk rationalities and the micro-politics of the care of the acutely ill in medicine was a moral evaluation founded upon the application of concepts of social worth common in the larger society (Roth 1972). Rescue was organised primarily around the timely and effective treatment of patients with one specific condition (Calnan *et al.* 2013). This reflected the primacy of specialism over generalism in hospital care, and highlighted an inbuilt discrimination against the major client group for acute care, that is, older patients with multiple comorbidities.

The primacy of the 'real emergency' in maternity
In maternity, the obstetric unit resource required protecting to ensure that those genuine emergencies were able to access specialist monitoring and medical treatment. Ensuring the safe crisis management of those already identified as acutely ill took priority over the safety and quality needs of women who were already housed on the obstetric units who had a potential risk of developing a complication:

> The midwife co-ordinator on the obstetric unit tells me about a recent shift she worked where she delayed accepting an admission from the antenatal ward on account of the needs of the women already housed on the obstetric unit. She had two women with twins in labour, all the labouring rooms were occupied and the waiting room was full of women waiting to be assessed. She said she perceived the unit was operating at 'maximum safety levels'. The woman who was waiting for the transfer had already been identified as unwell; while on the ward, her condition deteriorated quickly, she was found to be septic and needed a crash [emergency] caesarean section to deliver her baby. The midwife explains that she has been asked to write a statement to account for her decision. (Eastward, Field notes 6)

While the primacy of rescue enabled a timely response to the sudden obstetric emergency, detection of the slow drift of clinical deterioration in the antenatal and postnatal period was harder to manage. Boundary distinctions between the need for midwifery or obstetric-led care, and physiological and pathological trajectories were difficult to negotiate at times. This was particularly evident at Westward, where postnatally, women were often housed on the alongside midwifery unit as overspills from either the obstetric unit or postnatal ward. Medical staff tended to cross the boundary between the obstetric and alongside units only when an emergency call was put out. Securing a medical response for a woman whose condition was deteriorating slowly on the alongside unit was contingent on the presence of new symptoms which established a woman's' legitimacy for medical attention as a 'real emergency' (Dodier and Camus 1998):

> If you pull the emergency button immediately you have both the senior midwives from the obstetric unit or the doctors … and emergencies are acted on very quickly. But if you have someone who's a postnatal outlier needing to be reviewed, it may take a few hours before that woman gets reviewed … that kind of obstetric support is not here because it's set up for down in the postnatal ward. (Westward, Midwife, 4)

> We had a woman who had had a previous caesarean section, who had been having abdominal pains, not labour pains, generally feeling unwell and … we'd been waiting for her to be reviewed for a long, long time. In the end we decided to do a pre-eclampsia screen, it came back and her bloods were very abnormal. As soon as we had the proof of the bloods she was round next door as quick as a flash, but we'd been waiting eight, nine hours for a review. We'd been asking and escalating it [requesting a review and a step up in care]. (Westward, Midwife, 10)

Maternity services are structured around risk and women's trajectories to deal with possible crisis events. Boundaries are instituted through distinction practices. Gaining legitimate access to obstetric resources was difficult at times, particularly for women who were located outside the usual pathway through services and presented with a slow drift of deterioration, but were not yet at the point of collapse.

Discussion

In this chapter we suggest that Strauss *et al.*'s (1985) study of the social organisation of medical work offers a useful framework to theorise the complex care management of rescue, which remains relatively underdeveloped (Latimer 2014, Parker *et al.* 2000, Reiger 2011). We extend our lens of enquiry beyond the critical event of a patient's collapse to decision-making upstream. This enables us to explicate the linkages between such events and trajectories of care (Allen *et al.* 2004). Our focus on trajectories illuminates the physiological process of birth and the unfolding pathology of illness (and death). This frame provides a means for us to link the agency of those involved in organising the care of acutely ill patients with the wider socio-political factors beyond the clinic, such as governmentality and risk (Heyman 2010, Waring 2007), death brokering (Timmermans 2005) and the medicalisation of birth and death (De Vries 1981).

Since Jeffery's (1979) dichotomy of categories of good or interesting patients and 'normal rubbish' was criticised for being over-simplistic, research has tended to focus on the fluidity and interactional character of typifications in the emergency department (Dodier and Camus 1998, Hillman 2013, Hughes 1980, Nugus and Braithwaite 2010). While it is important to avoid overestimating the stability and influence of organisational bureaucratic structures and boundaries (Davies 2003), a sociology of practice needs to acknowledge the influence of organisational context, the structural elements, policies and relationships that are 'reestablished and reconstituted through work practices' (Timmermans 2006: 29). This chapter extends existing knowledge of categorisation practices in the emergency department to consider how patients' acute illness trajectories link to the ordering processes that occur in the socially structured conditions of the acute hospital ward. The chapter's novelty lies in its presentation of ethnographic material that illustrates relationships between the ideology of rescue, the perceived moral worth of patients, the handling of uncertainty in patients' acute illness trajectories and the intended and unintended consequences of risk technologies introduced to govern these trajectories for patient care.

While other studies investigating care in medical and maternity settings have highlighted how the labelling of patients adversely influences the way in which their care is organised, this chapter adds an important patient safety lens to the analysis. It adds to research showing how the management of risk and safety is politicised and applied locally (Annandale 1996, Brown and Calnan 2010, Scamell 2011, Tadd *et al.* 2011). Its specific contribution lies in insights generated over the often competing sets of medical, sociocultural, economic and political rationalities that face staff 'doing' patient safety. Reconciling quality, safety and efficiency is often difficult and requires constant trade-offs (Dixon-Woods *et al.* 2009, Nugus and Braithwaite 2010).

Not surprisingly, given recent policy emphasis on reducing the rates of avoidable death, which draw on cultural distinctions between the orderly and disorderly death (Bauman 1992, Bayatrizi 2008, Timmermans 2005), the rescue imperative provides a dominant organising frame across acute care. The logic of efficiency, effectiveness and safety in healthcare insists that cardiac arrests, an unexpected admission to ICU or death ought to be prevented. Risk technologies and audit data bring a degree of measurability to the management of critical illness, and help shape the organisation's generalisable knowledge about rescue work (Power 1997). An institutional audit culture that held practitioners accountable for their rescue work was particularly noticeable in maternity. Financial risk associated with failure to rescue overshadowed other risks (National Health Service Litigation Authority 2012). The management of rapidly unfolding clinical emergencies was arguably more tightly coupled to the outcome and the individuals involved in the rescue in maternity rather than in the medical settings, where clinical deterioration tended to occur over a longer period. In medical settings blame could be more easily diffused or relocated (Dixon-Woods *et al.* 2009).

Timmermans (1999) noted that the most outstanding social characteristics are the patient's age and the perceived seriousness of the illness with regard to the resuscitative effort. We note the significance of the elderly patient with complex conditions and the urgent maternal collapse in the broader construct of rescue trajectories. Our data support previous research suggesting that the delivery of acute hospital care is poorly designed to meet the safety needs of elderly patients with complex chronic conditions (Hillman *et al.* 2013, Latimer 2014, Tadd *et al.* 2011) and gate-keeping and legitimising practices in the maternity service contribute to problems accessing medical help (Kirkup 2015, McCourt *et al.* 2011). Our data add to the existing literature on the adverse consequences that can occur in the hospital for those who are categorised as not real emergencies (Dodier and Camus 1998) that is, 'neither in crisis nor completely stable' (Chapple 2010: 56), and the safety of outliers (Goulding *et al.* 2012). It extends the lens upstream from the construct of institutional death brokering (Timmermans 2005) to the active management of the physiological aspects of acute illness. Adverse events in patient safety are often not primarily due to human error at the ward level but are 'rather a systemic – or networked – consequence of the ways in which health work is related to cultures of management, governance and science' (Jensen 2008: 322).

Acknowledgements

The authors would like to thank Helen Rainey, Kylie Watson and Susanna Rance, who contributed to the research, and the reviewers for their helpful comments on earlier drafts of the chapter.

Nicola Mackintosh was funded by a National Institute for Health Research Patient Safety and Service Quality Research Fellowship (NIHR-PSSQRF-003). The research was supported by the National Institute for Health Research (NIHR) Collaboration for Leadership in Applied Health Research and Care South London at King's College Hospital NHS Foundation Trust. This chapter presents independent research funded by the NIHR. The views expressed are those of the authors and not necessarily those of the NHS, the NIHR or the Department of Health.

Notes

1   Number in brackets in the extracts refer to transcript descriptors.
2   In this obstetric emergency, the umbilical cord had been delivered prior to the baby so the first-line response necessitated taking pressure off the cord.

References

Allen, D., Griffiths, L. and Lyne, P. (2004) Understanding complex trajectories in health and social care provision, *Sociology of Health & Illness*, 26, 7, 1008–30.

Annandale, E. (1996) Working on the front-line: risk culture and nursing in the new NHS, *Sociological Review*, 44, 3, 416–51.

Bauman, Z. (1992) *Mortality, Immortality, and Other Life Strategies.* Stanford: Stanford University Press.

Bayatrizi, Z. (2008) *Life Sentences: The Modern Ordering of Mortality.* Toronto: University of Toronto Press.

Becker, H.S. (1993) How I learned what a crock was, *Journal of Contemporary Ethnography*, 22, 1, 28–8.

Bion, J.F. and Heffner, J.E. (2004) Challenges in the care of the acutely ill, *The Lancet*, 363, 9413, 970–7.

Bowker, G.C. and Star, S.L. (1999) *Sorting Things Out: Classification and its Consequences.* Cambridge: MIT Press.

Brown, P. and Calnan, M. (2010) The risks of managing uncertainty: the limitations of governance and choice, and the potential for trust, *Social Policy and Society*, 9, 1, 13–24.

Buist, M.D., Jarmolowski, E., Burton, P.R., Bernard, S.A., *et al.* (1999) Recognising clinical instability in hospital patients before cardiac arrest or unplanned admission to intensive care. A pilot study in a tertiary-care hospital, *Medical Journal of Australia*, 171, 1, 22–5.

Calnan, M., Tadd, W., Calnan, S., Hillman, A., *et al.* (2013) 'I often worry about the older person being in that system': exploring the key influences on the provision of dignified care for older people in acute hospitals, *Ageing and Society*, 33, 3, 465–85.

Chapple, H.S. (2010) *No Place for Dying: Hospitals and the Ideology of Rescue.* Walnut Creek: Left Coast Press.

Centre for Maternal and Child Enquiries (CMACE) (2011) Saving mothers' lives: reviewing maternal deaths to make motherhood safer: 2006–08. The eighth report on confidential enquiries into maternal deaths in the United Kingdom. *BJOG*, 118, 1–203.

Davies, C. (2003) Some of our concepts are missing: reflections on the absence of a sociology of organisations, *Sociology of Health & Illness*, 25, 3, 172–90.

De Vries, R. (1981) Birth and death: social construction at the poles of existence, *Social Forces*, 59, 4, 1074–93.

Degner, L.F. and Beaton, J.I. (1987) *Life and Death Decisions in Health Care.* Cambridge, New York and Philadelphia: Hemisphere.

Dingwall, R. (1977) 'Atrocity stories' and professional relationships, *Work and Occupations*, 4, 4, 371–96.

Dingwall, R. and Murray, T. (1983) Categorization in accident departments: 'good' patients, 'bad' patients and 'children', *Sociology of Health & Illness*, 5, 2, 127–48.

Dixon-Woods, M., Cavers, D., Agarwal, S., Annandale, E., *et al.* (2006) Conducting a critical interpretive synthesis of the literature on access to healthcare by vulnerable groups, *BMC Medical Research Methodology*, 6, 35, doi:10.1186/1471-2288-6-35.

Dixon-Woods, M., Suokas, A., Pitchforth, E. and Tarrant, C. (2009) An ethnographic study of classifying and accounting for risk at the sharp end of medical wards, *Social Science & Medicine*, 69, 3, 362–369.

Dodier, N. and Camus, A. (1998) Openness and specialisation: dealing with patients in a hospital emergency service, *Sociology of Health & Illness*, 20, 4, 413–4.

Emerson, R., Fretz, R. and Shaw, L. (1995) *Writing Ethnographic Fieldnote.*, Chicago: University of Chicago Press.

Glaser, B.G. (1998) *Doing Grounded Theory: Issues and Discussions.* Mill Valley: Sociology Press.

Goulding, L., Adamson, J., Watt, I. and Wright, J. (2012) Patient safety in patients who occupy beds on clinically inappropriate wards: a qualitative interview study with NHS staff, *British Medical Journal Quality and Safety*, 21, 3, 218–24.

Green, J. (2003) The ultimate challenge for risk technologies: controlling the accidental. In Summerton, J. and Berner, B. (eds) *Constructing Risk and Safety in Technological Practice.* London: Routledge.

Green, J. and Armstrong, D. (1993) Controlling the 'bed state': negotiating hospital organisation, *Sociology of Health & Illness*, 15, 3, 337–52.

Harrison, S. and Smith, C. (2004) Trust and moral motivation: redundant resources in health and social care?, *Policy and Politics*, 32, 3, 371–86.

Heyman, B. (2010) The concept of risk. In Heyman, B., Shaw, M., Alaszewski, A. and Titterton, M. (eds) *Risk, Safety and Clinical Practice. Health Care through the Lens of Risk*. Oxford: Oxford University Press.

Hillman, A. (2013) Why must I wait? The performance of legitimacy in a hospital emergency department, *Sociology of Health & Illness*, 36, 4, 485–99.

Hillman, A., Tadd, W., Calnan, S., Calnan, M., *et al.* (2013) Risk, governance and the experience of care, *Sociology of Health & Illness*, 35, 6, 939–55.

Hodgetts, T.J., Kenward, G., Vlackonikolis, I., Payne, S. *et al.* (2002) Incidence, location and reasons for avoidable in-hospital cardiac arrest in a district general hospital, *Resuscitation*, 54, 2, 115–23.

Hughes, D. (1980) The ambulance journey as an information generating process, *Sociology of Health & Illness*, 2, 2, 115–32.

Jeffery, R. (1979) Normal rubbish: deviant patients in casualty departments, *Sociology of Health & Illness*,1, 1, 90–107.

Jensen, C.B. (2008) Sociology, systems and (patient) safety: knowledge translations in healthcare policy, *Sociology of Health & Illness*, 30, 2, 309–24.

Johnson, J.C. (1990) *Selecting Ethnographic Informants*. Thousand Oaks: Sage.

King's Fund (2012) General service improvement tool. Available at http://www.kingsfund.org.uk/sites/-files/kf/field/field_related_document/Improving-safety-in-maternity-services-toolkit-service-improvement.pdf (accessed 15 November 2013).

Kirkup, B. (2015) *The report of the Morecambe Bay Investigation*. London: The Stationary Office.

Latimer, J. (2014) Nursing, the politics of organisation and meanings of care, *Journal of Research in Nursing*, 19, 7–8, 537–45.

McCourt, C., Rance, S., Rayment, J. and Sandall, J. (2011) Birthplace qualitative organisational case studies: how maternity care systems may affect the provision of care in different birth settings, Final report part, 6. Birthplace in England Research Programme.

Mackintosh, N. and Sandall, J. (2010) Overcoming gendered and professional hierarchies in order to facilitate escalation of care in emergency situations: the role of standardised communication protocols, *Social Science & Medicine*, 71, 9, 1683–6.

Mackintosh, N., Rainey, H. and Sandall, J. (2011) Understanding how rapid response systems may improve safety for the acutely ill patient: learning from the frontline, *BMJ Quality and Safety*, 21, 2, 135–44.

Mackintosh, N., Watson, K., Rance, S. and Sandall, J. (2013) Value of a modified early obstetric warning system (MEOWS) in managing maternal complications in the peripartum period: an ethnographic study, *BMJ Quality and Safety*, 23, 1, 26–34.

Mackintosh, N., Humphrey, C. and Sandall, J. (2014) The habitus of 'rescue' and its significance for implementation of rapid response systems in acute health care, *Social Science & Medicine*, 120, 233–42.

Mesman, J. (2008) *Uncertainty in Medical Innovation. Experienced Pioneers in Neonatal Care.* Basingstoke: Palgrave Macmillan.

National Audit Office (2013) *Maternity Services in England.* London: NAO.

National Confidential Enquiry into Patient Outcome and Death (NCEPOD) (2005) *An acute problem? A report of the National Confidential Enquiry into Patient Outcome and Death.* London: NCEPOD.

National Confidential Enquiry into Patient Outcome and Death (NCEPOD) (2012) *Time to intervene? A review of patients undergoing cardiopulmonary resuscitation as a result of an in-hospital cardiorespiratory arrest.* London: NCEPOD.

National Health Service Litigation Authority (2012) *Clinical Negligence Scheme for Trusts (CNST): maternity clinical risk management standards.* Version 1. London: NHSLA.

National Institute of Health and Clinical Excellence (NICE) (2007) *NICE clinical guideline 50. Acutely ill patients in hospital.* London: NICE.

National Patient Safety Agency (2007) *Safer care for the acutely ill patient: learning from serious incidents. PSO/5.* London: NPSA.

Nugus, P. and Braithwaite, J. (2010) The dynamic interaction of quality and efficiency in the emergency department: Squaring the circle?, *Social Science & Medicine*, 70, 4, 511–17.

Parker, G., Bhakta, P., Katbamna, S., Lovett, C., *et al.* (2000) Best place of care for older people after acute and during subacute illness: a systematic review, *Journal of Health Services Research and Policy*, 5, 3, 176–89.

Power, M. (1997) *The Audit Society: Rituals of Verification.* Oxford: Oxford University Press.

Rainey, H., Ehrich, K., Mackintosh, N. and Sandall, J. (2015) The role of patients and their relatives in 'speaking up' about their own safety – a qualitative study of acute illness, *Health Expectations*, 18, 3, 392–405.

Rance, S., Mccourt, C., Rayment, J., Mackintosh, N., *et al.* (2013) Women's safety alerts in maternity care: is speaking up enough?, *BMJ Quality and Safety*, 22, 4, 348–55.

Royal College of Midwives (2013) *State of maternity services report 2013.* London: RCM.

Reiger, K.M. (2011) 'Knights' or 'knaves'? Public policy, professional power, and reforming maternity services, *Health Care for Women International*, 32, 1, 2–22.

Ritchie, J. and Lewis, J. (eds) (2003) *Qualitative Research Practice: A Guide for Social Science Students and Researchers.* London: Sage.

Rittel, H. and Weber, M. (1973) Dilemmas in a general theory of planning, *Policy Sciences*, 4, 155–69.

Robson, C. (1993) *Real World Research: a Resource for Social Scientists.* Oxford: Blackwell.

Rockwood, K. and Hubbard, R. (2004) Frailty and the geriatrician, *Age and Ageing*, 33, 5, 429–30.

Roth, J.A. (1972) Some contingencies of the moral evaluation and control of clientele: the case of the hospital emergency service, *American Journal of Sociology*, 77, 5, 839–56.

Roth, W.-M. (2005) Making classifications (at) work: ordering practices in science, *Social Studies of Science*, 35, 6, 581–621.

Scamell, M. (2011) The swan effect in midwifery talk and practice: a tension between normality and the language of risk, *Sociology of Health & Illness*, 33, 7, 987–1001.

Schein, R.M., Hazday, N., Pena, M., Ruben, B.H., *et al.* (1990) Clinical antecedents to in-hospital cardiopulmonary arrest, *Chest*, 98, 6, 1388–92.

Smith, G., Osgood, V. and Crane, S. (2002) ALERT – a multiprofessional course in care of the acutely ill adult patient, *Resuscitation*, 52, 3, 281–86.

Smith, V. (2007) Ethnographies of Work and the Work of Ethnographers. In Atkinson, P., Coffey, A., Delamont, S., Lofland, J. *et al.* (eds) *Handbook of Ethnography.* Los Angeles: Sage.

Strauss A.L., Fagerhaugh, S., Suczek, B. and Wiener, C. (1985) *Social Organisation of Medical Work.* Chicago: University of Chicago Press.

Strauss, A.L., Fagerhaugh, S., Suczek, B. and Wiener, C. (1997) *Social Organisation of Medical Work*, 2nd edn. Chicago: University of Chicago Press.

Suokas, A.K. (2010) *Early Warning Systems and the Organisational Dynamics of Standardisation.* PhD thesis, Leicester, University of Leicester.

Tadd, W., Hillman, A., Calnan, S., Calnan, M., *et al.* (2011) Right place – wrong person: dignity in the acute care of older people, *Quality in Ageing and Older Adults*, 12, 1, 33–43.

Timmermans, S. (1999) *Sudden Death and the Myth of CPR.* Philadelphia: Temple University Press.

Timmermans, S. (2005) Death brokering: constructing culturally appropriate deaths, *Sociology of Health & Illness*, 27, 7, 993–1013.

Timmermans, S. (2006) *Postmortem. How Medical Examiners Explain Suspicious Deaths.* Chicago, The University of Chicago Press.

Tsoukas, H. (1997) The tyranny of light: the temptations and the paradoxes of the information society, *Futures*, 29, 9, 827–43.

Vassy, C. (2001) Categorisation and micro-rationing: access to care in a French emergency department, *Sociology of Health & Illness*, 23, 5, 615–32.

Walsh, D. (2006) Subverting the assembly-line: childbirth in a free-standing birth centre, *Social Science & Medicine*, 62, 6, 1330–40.

Waring, J. (2007) Adaptive regulation or governmentality: patient safety and the changing regulation of medicine, *Sociology of Health & Illness*, 29, 2, 163–79.

Winters, B.D., Weaver, S.J., Pfoh, E.R., Yang, T., *et al.* (2013) Rapid-response systems as a patient safety strategy: a systematic review, *Annals of Internal Medicine*, 158, 5, 417–25.

6

Sensemaking and the co-production of safety: a qualitative study of primary medical care patients
Penny Rhodes, Ruth McDonald, Stephen Campbell, Gavin Daker-White and Caroline Sanders

Introduction

Studies investigating primary care patients' understandings of safety have been largely concerned with how patients define errors in their care and reveal that the scope of patient reported harms and their causes tends to be wider than that recognised by healthcare professionals (e.g. Burgess *et al.* 2012, Kuzel *et al.* 2004). However, patient safety is broader than absence of error (Amalberti *et al.* 2011), not all errors result in harm and not all harm is the result of error (Vincent *et al.* 2013).

Recent sociological work has exposed the ways in which 'medical errors' and 'safety' are continually and contingently re/defined and re/negotiated by practitioners (e.g. Hor *et al.* 2010, Yeung and Dixon-Woods 2010). Thus, safety can be perceived as an on-going, practical accomplishment of health professionals interacting with each other, their resources, spaces and tasks in the course of their work (e.g. McDonald *et al.* 2006, Mesman 2009). More recently there has been recognition of the role of patients and their friends and family in the co-production of healthcare safety (Doherty and Saunders 2013, Hor *et al.* 2013, Hrisos and Thomson 2013). This means that, as 'safety' involves professionals and relevant lay people in a re/negotiation and re/definition process, it can never be 'fully mapped out *a priori*' through prospective design (Iedema *et al.* 2006: 1210).

Patients' perspectives and experiences of safety are likely to vary in different contexts. Existing work has tended to be based on hospital or hospice settings. However, primary care is an important domain for researching patients' perspectives, as it provides direct access to medical professionals. As a first contact point, many consultations are mainly initiated by patients, and medical expertise in primary care is of a generalist nature unlike for example, more specialised hospital care. Although surveillance has increased in this setting (Chew-Graham *et al.* 2013), for conditions which are not subject to financial incentives, care may be less systematised (McDonald *et al.* 2013). Yet little sociologically informed work has examined this topic.

Sensemaking and safety

Various studies have used Weick's (1995) concept of sensemaking as a lens through which to view professional behaviours and actions in relation to patient safety. For example, Doherty

The Sociology of Healthcare Safety and Quality, First Edition. Edited by Davina Allen, Jeffrey Braithwaite, Jane Sandall and Justin Waring. Chapters © 2016 The Authors. Book Compilation © 2016 Foundation for the Sociology of Health & Illness/Blackwell Publishing Ltd.

and Saunders (2013) have examined elective surgical patients' sensemaking and the implications of this for the co-construction of safety. According to Weick, sensemaking is the process by which people enact their environments. It requires an articulation of the unknown in order to make sense of complexity, 'turning circumstances into a situation that is comprehended explicitly in words and serves as a springboard to action' (Weick 2005: 409). Sensemaking is a social process with individuals interacting with people and objects to interpret their surroundings. Whilst some have depicted this as a cognitive information processing activity (Weick 1995), more recently there has been an emphasis on the emotional and embodied aspects of sensemaking (Cunliffe and Coupland 2012). As we discuss later, not everybody has a fully formed set of views on safety in primary care. Indeed, for many, an assumption that primary healthcare settings are safe (Fotaki 2014) may indicate lack of prior reflection on the topic of their safety. Asking people to talk about their experiences and perceptions in this context is a way of tapping into and prompting their sensemaking processes. Sensemaking is about action, as much as it is about talk. Yet being able to articulate one's perceptions is a key part of the sensemaking process.

Sensemaking has implications not just for how we see the world around us, but also for our understanding of who we are. To maintain our self-esteem and approval of others we must tell stories which fit with the wider environment. Individuals are not social dopes but they make sense of the world in the context of their personal life and experiences, which means that they may be subject to 'taken for granted' beliefs about the 'natural order' of things. In the context of knowledge asymmetry, there may be a readiness to defer to medical professionals. A breach or disruption to normal activities, which means that available cues and frameworks are insufficient to facilitate immediate understanding, is likely to prompt sensemaking of a more episodic nature (Weick 2012). This has been seen to occur when individuals spend time as hospital inpatients, a setting which is largely unfamiliar to them, and where control has to be surrendered to medical protocols and treatment procedures. Doherty and Saunders (2013: 35) describe the surgical patients in their study as vulnerable and uncertain, passive and subordinate making 'excuses to mitigate any negative inferences that could be attributed to clinicians' actions'. Compared with hospital settings, people have much more experience of primary medical care encounters, with visits to the local general practice following routines and patterns, which are to some extent predictable. The nature of primary care then, arguably offers more opportunities for action than is the case in secondary care.

In this chapter, therefore, we ask how individuals make sense of their experiences of primary medical care and how that sensemaking shapes and reshapes their conceptualisation of safety. We also ask to what extent this resonates with findings (Doherty and Saunders 2013) about the way hospital patients engage in sensemaking and co-production of safety.

Methods

Ethics approval was provided by the Proportionate Review Sub-Committee of the National Research Ethics Service (NRES) Committee London – City & East, REC reference: 12/LO/1588. Participants were initially recruited through five general practices in the northwest of England. We aimed to have a maximum variation sample according to age, education level, carer status, socioeconomic and ethnic background. We deliberately over-sampled for people with multiple long-term conditions, due to increased vulnerability to patient safety incidents (Scobie 2010).

Fourteen men and 24 women were interviewed and age ranged from 18 to 78 years (60% over 50 years). Fifteen people were recruited through their practice, the remainder through snowballing. Participants were registered with 19 practices across the northwest of England. Participants had visited their GP an average of 5 times (range = 1–12). Twenty-five respondents had one or more long term conditions, 12 of whom had more than one condition.

Interviews were mostly conducted in participants' homes, depending on preference; and all participants signed a consent form. All interviews were conducted by the same person (PR), lasted between 30 minutes and 2 hours, were audio-recorded and transcribed. Participants were asked basic socio-demographic details (age, marital status, length of time at current practice, number of visits to practice in past 12 months, presence of long term conditions). A topic guide was developed and interviews began with broad questions, (e.g. 'If I mention patient safety in general practice, what would you think of?'). We deliberately did not frame questions around formal concepts such as 'error' or 'harm', and, in order to elicit their own understandings, participants were enabled to introduce topics they considered relevant. Patient initiated topics included access, continuity, privacy and doctors' manner. As it became apparent that perceptions of quality and safety were often interlinked, later interviews sought to unpick the distinction. Where there was ambiguity, the interviewer sought clarification.

All transcripts were anonymised with participants identified by gender (M/F) and assigned a unique identification number. Transcripts were entered into NVivo10 (qualitative data software package; Brisbane, QS International) and analysed thematically and iteratively, drawing on grounded theory techniques to generate open codes which were constantly compared across cases (Corbin and Strauss 2008). We used memos and team discussions to distil the core themes and to identify and discuss unusual cases. Initial coding was carried out by one author (PR) and selected transcripts were read and coded by additional authors to identify key themes. Sixty four first order codes were categorised within seven main themes comprising: physical, psychological and interpersonal safety; medical safety; communication safety; systems safety; timely access; holistic care and relationship continuity; flexibility in the interpretation of rules. Through further analysis and discussion, these initial themes were distilled into three core themes: (i) trust and psycho-social aspects of professional-patient relationships; (ii) choice, continuity, access and the temporal underpinnings for safety and (iii) organisational and systems-level tensions constraining safety. The main findings in relation to these core themes have been reported elsewhere (Rhodes *et al.* 2014, 2015). However, for this chapter, we have reanalysed the data using Weick's framework to understand sensemaking around primary care patient safety amongst primary care patients.

Findings

The narratives in policy and academic literatures about safety in primary care tend to focus on designing and maintaining safe systems and disseminating guidelines aimed at reducing error. The accounts of patients suggested a somewhat different conceptualisation of safety, as we describe below.

Sensemaking and the articulation of safety
When initially asked how they understood safety in primary care, people were unsure how to respond and would throw the question back:

What do you mean by safety issues? (F.25)
I don't know what we mean by patient safety. (F.06)

Many responses seemed to be suggestive of the work to make sense of this concept that they had not previously thought about in any depth:

> To be honest you never really think about it, do you, until asked. (F.31)
> I'd never thought about the safety implications. (F.32)

First thoughts were often about the risks posed by other patients or features of the physical environment, such as dangerous stairs:

> I think there's a safety issue around other patients actually as well … it has a very cramped waiting room and sometimes people are coughing and spluttering, et cetera, and, if you're immuno-suppressed, you wouldn't necessarily want to sit next to them. And also, when people get very uptight in a GP surgery, it can be a bit unnerving. (F.18)

> Before my practice moved to where they are now, they were in an old house with a very, very steep a staircase with very short treads. It was designed to suit people in the 1830s when people were much smaller. (F.05)

Medical competence, seen as the effective application of abstract, encoded knowledge (Nettleton *et al.* 2008), was considered a prerequisite for safety:

> Top – safety in terms of my definition, you know, professional competence, the current practical knowledge and peer reviews of performance of that sort – if all that is embraced in safety, then it's at the top – more important than accessibility, length of time you've got to wait for an appointment, much, much more important than that. The reason that I go to the doctor is because I trust that he is able to deal with me confidently. (M.01)

Participants found it difficult to disentangle safety from quality. Many aspects of care or service appreciated in terms of quality were also aspects that made them feel safe. Systems for allocating appointments on a 'first come, first served' basis, for example, were thought to be unfair on the grounds that not all patients are able to take equal advantage of them, and became unsafe when patients in genuine need of rapid access were unable to obtain it, as happened to one patient who was subsequently admitted to hospital as an emergency.

Accessibility embraced more than the ease or difficulty of obtaining an appointment. References to accessibility included the extent to which patients felt confident in approaching the service in the first place, what one person referred to as 'approachability'. 'Approachability' included references to the physical environment, and the manner and attitude of reception staff (Swinglehurst *et al.*, 2011):

> Approachability, meaning a welcoming environment, a good receptionist, an efficient process of booking in, a good appointment system, a variety of general practitioners. (F.06)

As we have written elsewhere, participants' perspectives on safety within primary care comprised psycho-social as well as physical dimensions (Rhodes *et al.* 2015). Psycho-social safety is essentially a relational concept generated both from people's expectations about how a forthcoming relationship might unfold and the interaction within that unfolding relationship, which can reinforce or confound expectations. Many participants for example, described a need for doctors to take time in a context of patient vulnerability:

> So I don't want to be with someone that just palms me off, because they haven't got the time … for someone who comes in and is projecting as fragile and vulnerable. (F.25)

Sensemaking from experience: reflecting on safety in practice
Although people often had difficulty thinking about safety in the abstract, they were more confident in describing specific situations in which they had felt unsafe:

> What was handled badly was him not taking my daughter being ill seriously … And it meant that I felt that I couldn't go back to the GPs because I would just be told, 'Well, what are you worried about?'
>
> Interviewer: So you felt you had no option but to go the hospital route?
>
> Respondent: Yes, and that's what my friends were telling me, 'You'll just have to take her to hospital'. So I felt kind of unsupported, if you like, as a result. (F.07) (Mother whose child was eventually diagnosed at the hospital with a form of encephalitis)
>
> The one time I did see him before the cancer diagnosis he had me in and out of the surgery that fast that I didn't even manage to bring up the reason I'd gone in. (F.07) (woman with mental illness and cancer)

People often drew on their own experiences to substantiate or validate their views. For example, one woman justified her lack of confidence in GPs in general by describing a catalogue of examples of (in her view) poor and unsafe care. A succession of different doctors and their failure to take her concerns seriously compromised both her physical and psychological safety, and undermined her confidence in GPs in general. The negative consequences extended beyond the problem that was misdiagnosed to future relationships with GPs and future consulting behaviour:

> I knew there was a problem (and) I needed to go and see a specialist but that still didn't happen. [It was] 'Let's just try you on these tablets'. Because I knew it wasn't an infection, (but) they kept saying for eighteen months I had an ear infection … I had to actually spell it out to them, that's what I feel … which worries me for somebody else … I'm not a pushy person, but the only times I've got referred for something like that is when I've become a bit pushy … and I've said, 'Look I've been coming since then, I've tried this and that and it's (not any better)'. (F.21)

One respondent had moved practices due to negative experiences and problems with access, and described the reasons why he felt safe in the new practice:

> Why I feel safe … well, the main concern about going to places like that would be, you know, spread of a virus, maybe, or something like that, so it's always clean, you know, people are prompted to wash their hands when they go in, you know, the gel. People, like my father, he's in a wheelchair, you know, he's got a ramp provided, stair lifts, people look after you if you need anything, straight away, you know, one of the receptionists will come out and say, do you need anything? So the whole environment is, you know,

and it is a very small house if you go in, you know, it's not very clinical, it's, like, a house basically. (M.32)

Although a good physician will have the ability to make patients feel both psychologically and physically safe, patients recognised that these two dimensions draw on different qualities and skills and not all doctors will be proficient in both: a doctor's poor interpersonal skills, for example, might be balanced by greater technical competence. Some patients therefore had preferred doctors for different types of problem:

> (At) my previous practice, there were two doctors. One of whom was lovely, and everybody wanted to see, and the other was grumpy and nobody wanted to see. So, if you wanted to see the first doctor, you might have to wait weeks. To see this other doctor, you could see him any time, but I came to the conclusion that, actually, the one that nobody liked was a better diagnostician. (M.30)

However, in prioritising one (physical or psychological safety), patients could compromise the other, either wittingly (as in the case of the man who was reluctant to consult a GP about his smokers' cough because he knew it to be self-inflicted) or unwittingly. An example of the latter can be illustrated by the case of a woman who persisted with her familiar GP until she was eventually diagnosed with cancer by a new doctor. In reflecting back on these events, she felt her original GP had misattributed her symptoms of cancer to the natural processes of aging. Some participants distinguished between feeling and being safe, in the recognition that a sense of psychological security could be misleading and trust misplaced:

> I don't know if that's, you know, in the end, more safe or not, because, if you trust somebody more, you might not check them properly, (check) what they do … But you feel safe, definitely. (M.32)

Patients had to balance not only the different dimensions of safety but to weigh them against other priorities and social imperatives. Safety, for patients, was not necessarily always their top priority, and their decisions may not always have been considered 'safe' from the perspective of health professionals. Examples where other social imperatives took precedence include a Muslim woman with diabetes who chose to fast during Ramadan against her doctor's advice, and a man who delayed visiting the GP about his abdominal pain because he could not take time off work.

Perceptions of safety were thus open to multiple interpretations, and achieving safe care was often a matter of negotiation between patient and GP. In some cases, patients tried to persuade GPs of their own (rival) interpretation: for example, the person with a misdiagnosed ear condition (quoted above) who refused more antibiotics and insisted on a hospital referral. Negotiation, however, was not always attempted or successful, and, in other cases, patients bypassed the GP by contacting the hospital directly, simply ignored what they perceived to be unsafe advice and/or treatment, or sought help elsewhere by consulting a different GP:

> There was one time I got home and, when I realised, I was so angry because I'd said to them I'd had these tablets and they'd been no good and they'd made me feel ill, and they'd actually prescribed the very same tablets … I didn't take the tablets because I knew they made me feel ill and they didn't work. (F.21)

I've been to see a GP in my practice who doesn't know me and he's said something, and I knew that wasn't the way to treat somebody who'd got renal failure and so I just ignored what he said. (F.18)

Participants were often drawing attention to the emotions engendered in related healthcare encounters:

And I remember I came back to see her before she left and, you know, there was some actual physical contact. She put her hand on my shoulder. I can't quite remember whether I actually hugged her, but you know, I really felt like she really cared about what was going to happen to me, and there was that human element. It wasn't that I'm a little minion on a conveyor belt through your practice. (F.25)

But then on the day that I was at my worst, literally it was at the worst you could imagine, she said to me … I'm going to close the book on your physical health because there's nothing wrong with you, and I'm going to open the book on your psychological because it's all psychologically based. So I was like in tears at that point … I could easily have taken my life at that (point), because I was at my lowest. Because I knew something wasn't right and this woman was just ignoring me … I feel so angry about … even to this day. (F.26)

Trust was not just engendered at cognitive level but at an emotional and affective level. And, for many people, it was this emotional response that was most potent in inspiring more generalised confidence in a doctor's medical knowledge and skill. When people felt safe at a psycho-social level, they also felt more confident in the doctor's medical capabilities to deal with their physical health concerns. Feeling safe, in the sense of avoidance or minimisation of emotional harm was important to patients, but is not articulated in policy guidance and represents a very different conceptualisation of safety from that espoused in official safety discourse:

I would say it was fine, but not personal at all, you know, you didn't feel that connection.

Interviewer: Do you think that connection is just a, sort of, something you like, a quality of service issue or do you think it might have or had safety implications?

Good question that – you feel more safe, I don't know if it has a safety implication, but you feel, as a person, you feel more safe, you feel you trust the other person more. (M.32)

'Feeling safe' embraced feelings of psychological and emotional as well as physical safety. The following comment typified the views of many:

I think your care and approach is just as much part of what you are expecting from a GP or any doctor, really, as the actual medical judgement. (F.07)

Others commented:

They (GPs) don't realise how we have to psych ourselves up to go in the first place. (F.25)

Sometimes it's not an easy thing to go in there … because sometimes I feel like I'm wasting their time and feeling guilty about being there, that's how I felt. (F.18)

Participants reported developing strategies, based on previous experience, to protect their psycho-social safety. These strategies resonate with previous research on help-seeking and reasons for delayed diagnosis (Smith *et al.* 2005), and included waiting until they have a concern less likely to be judged trivial and appending the 'trivial' concern to the more weighty concern:

> And I felt, well, those problems were small, so I'm going … you know, I will come with three small problems, because one of those problems seems significant …
>
> Interviewer: Am I putting words into your mouth by saying, if you think something's trivial you won't go, but you will take it once you get something else as well?
>
> Yeah, as a bolt-on to perhaps a more significant thing … And I got a kind of brusque kind of, you know, I long for a time when you don't come with a long list. (F.25)

Additional strategies included avoiding contact with doctors from whom they have had a poor reception in the past:

> A long time ago, I went with quite serious anxiety problems, and he actually said, 'Pull yourself together', and sent me back to work. Obviously I never saw him again. (F.31)

Seeking continuity with a familiar and trusted GP was also a common strategy which is reported in detail elsewhere (Rhodes *et al.* 2014). For example, one respondent talked about the difficulties of managing to get an appointment with a doctor who they had already consulted with, and with whom they wanted a further consultation. The interviewer clarified whether this was perceived to be a safety issue:

> Interviewer: Right, do you think that's mainly a convenience issue or do you think there are safety implications?
>
> I think they're safety implications … I don't necessarily mind which doctor I see, but if I've started to see one about a particular condition, then I'd like to continue to see that person, because then they have a better picture about how things are progressing, or whether they're progressing and I don't have to do the whole story again and spend time talking to them for too long to tell them the story, so I'd prefer to see the same person. (F.29)

Participants were also anxious about their own performance during the consultation and concerned that they would not be able to express themselves adequately or understand and remember what was said to them:

> Not everybody explains themselves well, some people are nervous, it's like visiting a lawyer … you're frightened about the language they speak and I think it's the same with a lot of people with doctors. (F.10)
>
> When you go to the doctor, it's like you know you've only got 5 mins and you've got to get it out, you know. The number of times you come away and you think, Oh no, I didn't mention that part about it or something, you know! (F.07)

Proactive patients and the co-production of safety

The degree to which individuals had reflected on the need to actively intervene to contribute to safe or safer encounters varied widely across our participants. Greater awareness of the risks came with greater exposure and responses indicated that patients' experiences changed the nature of their use of primary care services (see also Elder *et al.* 2005). People who were frequent users of health services (both younger and older respondents) had generally become more knowledgeable about the way they operated than those with less experience. Additionally, they were better able to negotiate the interface between self-care and formal, professional care, and more alert to safety risks and aware of measures to guard against them (cf. Hernan 2014). They therefore tended to be less complacent and perceived themselves better able to take proactive measures to protect themselves: examples included checking prescriptions and communications between hospital and surgery; alerting unfamiliar health practitioners to specific risks, such as adverse reactions to specific medication; becoming knowledgeable about their own condition/s and vulnerabilities; finding out about different treatment options; challenging clinicians' decisions and practice procedures. One couple, both with serious co-morbidity, explained:

Husband: When (wife) has got a particular problem, we generally know what the solution to this problem is. We've obviously got to go to the GP, we can't write prescriptions out ourselves, we don't have any formal medical training, it's just experience, really. So, when we go to the GP, it's pretty easy to spot whether they know what they are talking about, rather than just guessing at stuff.

Wife: They're receptive to our knowledge and we respect their knowledge.

Husband: We are very fortunate in that we are reasonably well educated and we kind of know how the system works and that we have been in it for a long time. (F.08, M.09 joint interview)

As the extract demonstrates, the ability to take a proactive role was dependent on patients' expertise and knowledge accumulated over time, the social distance between doctor and patient, and patients' self-confidence to question and be assertive. In consequence, some patients were more empowered and more capable of adopting a proactive role than others:

> I do feel I have to … sort of lead them, be clued up, be pushy and it's almost like I feel like there are trigger words that you have to say. (F.21)

Safety, and the capacity for agency (individuals acting independently and making their own free choices), were therefore unequally distributed, and allusion to these fundamental inequalities was a common theme in many of the interviews. The couple quoted above, for example, commented:

Husband: We have friends who have not had that level of experience or expertise and they definitely get a worse deal from their doctors than if you are able to present your argument or present your case, and I think that is important, you know. This question of safety does depend a lot on the patient, and maybe there is a need to have a system that isn't so patient-dependent.

Interviewer: So, you feel you are adequately informed and involved in discussions about what you are going to have?

Wife: Yes, we are not sure if it is because of who we are and how we talk to doctors … I wouldn't have that same trust, if I was less informed and less able myself.

Husband: Or less experienced.

Wife: That's exactly the problem – if you are not aware, you just go ahead and do whatever, you don't check. (F.08, M.09 joint interview)

In one person's view, it was this presumption of safety which posed the greatest barrier to patients taking a more active role:

[Patients] need to be more aware of health and safety around them, and not presume that things are not going to happen. (M.33)

Participants sometimes indicated that they downplayed or forgave mistakes because acknowledging the possibility of unsafe care might have troublesome consequences. For example, one man described his experiences of repeatedly lost test results which he downplayed stating that he did not feel able to move practice anyway, because of difficulty of travelling to a more distant practice and the fact that none of doctors could speak Urdu, the only language of his wife. However, in the following example, this respondent indicated that repeated exposure to problems over time made it increasingly difficult to ignore them, prompting action to mitigate harm and perceived threats to safe care. This suggests that for some patients there may be a threshold for action, although this is likely to vary between patients and contexts:

I think it was gradually, you know, when you go somewhere and you're not happy with the service, but you try to placate yourself, and you try to make yourself believe that it was just a one off, and you've got to give somebody the benefit of the doubt, they might be having a bad day, something like that. So you're continually doing that, and then you reach a point when you think, I've reached saturation level now, and I'm not going to take this kind of attitude. (F.16)

Participants often indicated they were vaguely aware of changes in procedures regulating quality and safety; however, there was general lack of clarity about the nature of the changes or understanding of the rationale underpinning them. Much of what was said indicated that the changes, although designed to enhance quality and safety, were often experienced as obstacles.

The invisibility or opacity of much of the formal architecture of safety meant that it was inaccessible to patient scrutiny or evaluation, leaving patients with only a general sense of more tightly governed practice. Patients expected and assumed GPs would adhere to the tenets of safe practice, but were ambivalent about the erosion of GPs' discretionary space (c.f. Horlick-Jones 2005). Whereas policymakers see the promotion of guidelines as encouraging safe practice, if anything, diminished opportunities for discretion were thought to undermine, rather than promote, safety, with standard rules and procedures: (i) operating as constraints on the provision of individualised care, and disadvantaging for some patients, (ii) seen as a protection more for health professionals than patients, and (iii) making it difficult to judge when doctors were speaking or acting on their own accounts or in accordance with the officially prescribed view:

They just follow the rules and regulations and guidelines … and can't be allowed to slightly deviate and use a bit of common sense and be credited with having a bit of intelligence. (F.23)

They are frightened of being sued … And, sadly, that is what leads to a lot of the bureaucracy … They're given a script and they follow it, they're scared of moving off the script. (M.09)

I feel that they've got their targets and that seems to override their own thoughts… And it is very hard, because they are … paid according to those targets, to know how much they are just pushing it because they have to or whether they really do believe in it.

Interviewer: So, what you are saying is that it distorts.
… . having a meaningful discussion with your medical practitioner. (F.07)

In participants' opinions, many of the visible bulwarks of safety – home visits by a familiar doctor, continuing personal relationships with specific practitioners and engagement with patients as individuals – have been steadily eroded, to be replaced by a less visible or accessible framework of standards and protocols.

Discussion

The accounts of patients in our study suggested that what makes them feel safe is often very different from the sorts of things which focus the attention of policymakers and clinicians. Patients' accounts suggested that safety was not something 'out there' that could be readily identified, codified in guidelines and measured, but in many cases was an emergent product of interaction between people, and between people and their environment. Safety was understood, not as a unified, objective and apolitical conception of what it means to be safe, but as a fluid, contingent, contestable, and negotiable accomplishment. Patients found it much easier to draw on experience when making sense of safety than to conceptualise and articulate it in abstract terms. At the same time, when questioned, some participants began to reflect and articulate aspects of primary care (such as approachability) which were important to them in terms of making them feel safe.

Safety, for patients, was multi-dimensional and the different dimensions could variously complement, reinforce, undermine, compete or conflict with each other, depending on the situation. The constitution of safe care was, therefore, inherently unstable – what might be considered safe in some circumstances, might be considered less safe or unsafe in others. It was also personal: one person's conception of what it means to be safe might be different from that of another, different in different contexts and, crucially, different from that of health practitioners. Achieving safe care was therefore a matter of individual negotiation between patient and practitioner.

Patients' understandings recognised that the dimensions of safety might be in tension with each other and with other priorities at the personal, practice and wider local and national level. Patients were aware of a need for difficult trade-offs at the level of individual patients' strategies (e.g. accepting an early appointment with an unfamiliar GP or waiting longer for an appointment with a familiar GP) and broader policy (e.g. prioritising accessibility, in terms of length of consultation, over flexibility in matching timings to individual patients' needs), and that the imposition of standard rules would create 'winners' and 'losers'. Standard rules, such as those regulating access, were often perceived to be neither fair nor safe and the safest systems to be those which offered some flexibility.

We did not observe patients and have to rely on their accounts, but many reported employing informal strategies to protect their own safety. Their strategies were shaped by a more expansive interpretation of safety than that which inspires formal safety schemes, and were constrained, not just by limited knowledge of the risks to which they might be exposed but by aspects of service organisation and wider policy, and might not always be deemed 'safe' from the perspective of health professionals. Weick (1995) observes that a sense of powerlessness can account for the maintenance of faith and trust in safety systems because the alternative is to face anxiety and fear without any means of addressing the source. On the whole, patients presumed that there were systems in place to protect their physical safety but had little or no knowledge of what they were or how they operated. Given the invisibility or opacity of much of the technical apparatus of safety, it is not surprising that participants' accounts often gave greater prominence to the more accessible psycho-social dimension of safety in which they were both more knowledgeable and more proficient in taking an active role.

Sensemaking encompasses presumption and entails actively connecting the abstract and concrete in a way that draws on experience. Experiences which involve a breach in one's presumptions (such as interactions with unfriendly receptionist or incompetent doctors) appeared to prompt reappraisal and reshaping. Whilst sensemaking is retrospective (i.e. people try to make sense of what happened in the past), it has implications for the present and the future. In particular, patients' presumptions are important since they are a basis for future action (or avoidance of action). Several patients reported being proactive and 'on their guard' as a result of prior negative experiences. At the same time, other presumptions (around doctors' behaviours towards smokers, or their views of some consultations/concerns as being trivial) appeared to be based on an appreciation that particular identities (the smoker, the NHS resource waster, the hypochondriac) are viewed in a negative light. To some extent this resonates with the concept of 'identity threat' (Coyle 1999) which involves a challenge to personal identity as a result of experiences which are felt to be disempowering and devaluing. For our participants, the way that they made sense of things resulted in them taking action in anticipation of events, rather than undergoing such experiences.

Sensemaking organises flux. But participants' accounts often described the routine and the familiar, which appears to reflect the fact that most of the people interviewed were experienced users of primary care. Rather than viewing doctors as powerful and trusting them unconditionally, many participants reported using judgments, often based on prior experience, to structure their interactions with doctors. This contrasts with Doherty and Saunders's (2013: 35) findings that 'patients generally constructed themselves in a subordinate trusting role, where they should follow the rules laid down by clinicians, the people they believe are the most qualified to make the decisions because they have the requisite technical knowledge.' Doctors in our study were constructed as having to follow 'rules and regulations', being 'scared of moving off the script' and having 'targets that seem to override their own thoughts'.

Despite this, participants also displayed a high degree of trust in many cases, in a way which resonates with Giddens's (1990) ideas about trust in abstract systems. Such trust may be reinforced or reduced as part of our interactions which form our concrete experiences. Of course, such trust occurs within relationships characterised by inequality, given the gap between medical professionals and patients in terms of medical knowledge. At the same time, patients with chronic conditions are likely to develop expertise about their condition and, as our data show, do not necessarily defer to medical opinion in all cases. However, patients also appeared constrained as a result of their awareness of the rules of interaction with their doctor. Their fear of being judged by them and reports of continuing to consult (as opposed to going elsewhere) despite reservations, suggest that patients do not always take action to avoid unnecessary harm.

Weick *et al.* (2005) have described how health professionals engage in labelling and categorisation as part of a process of making sense of a potentially chaotic situation. This enables imposition of diagnostic labels which imply plausible treatments. Our findings suggest that patients also engage in this process, labelling and pigeonholing doctors, receptionists and premises and such labelling carries implications for action.

This means that whilst both groups engage in sensemaking, the sense made differs between them. This is understandable, but it has important implications. Patients do not, necessarily, voice concerns in consultations, but a lack of trust in a doctor's abilities, a fear of being judged or presumptions about guidelines constraining doctors can lead patients to ignore or avoid medical advice, which may have consequences for patient safety. Whilst the patients in our study appeared less passive than the hospital patients studied by Doherty and Saunders (2013), in both cases, accounts highlight the gulf between clinicians and patients in the way that sense is made of interactions and contexts. In addition, Doherty and Saunders (2013: 35) suggest that 'guided sensemaking is required to enable shared understanding and more reliable decision making'. This process involves clinicians being more interactive, rather than didactic and takes time. In the context of primary care, which has traditionally been characterised by relational continuity, the potential exists for clinicians to pick up on cues and broaden the scope of noticing and labelling beyond the availability of medically formulated mental models. Interactions as part of an ongoing relationship provide an opportunity over time, to significantly bridge the gap between the sense that is made by patients and clinicians. This is not a suggestion that we should return to a mythical 'golden age' when such gaps did not exist. Furthermore, as highlighted by some of our patients, locums or other unfamiliar doctors can spot things that the patient's 'usual' doctor has missed. However, the shift in emphasis away from relational continuity with a single doctor (Hill *et al.* 2011) means that the potential for the development of shared understanding as part of an ongoing relationship is diminished.

Conclusions

Our study explored primary care patients' sensemaking, with an explicit focus on safety. Contrary to the findings in a recent study examining sensemaking amongst hospital surgical patients, we found participants were often proactive in taking action to protect themselves. The somewhat routinised and predictable nature of the primary medical care consultation, which is very different from 'one off' inpatient spells meant that patients had a stock of accumulated knowledge and experience to inform their actions. This also seemed to equip them with a wider repertoire of potential options for action. Participants' accounts underscore the salience of a psycho-social dimension to harm and the importance of psycho-social safety, which can exist independently of any association with physical harm or functional impairment. This highlights the need for a much broader conceptualisation of what it means to be safe. Despite increased recognition of the importance of psychological and emotional harm in healthcare settings (e.g. Burgess *et al.* 2012, Kuzel *et al.* 2004), conceptualisations of harm remain largely confined within a biomedical focus on functional impairment (World Health Organisation 2009).

Much of the writing from the patient safety literature has focused on minimising risks and hazards drawing on lessons from the aviation industry. The result has often been a focus on rules and checklists intended to prevent error (Waring 2009). This approach tends to neglect the different ways in which safety is conceptualised by different groups within such systems (Brown 2008). Yet even among health professionals and within organisations, there are likely to be multiple voices and perspectives on this issue (e.g. Currie *et al.* 2009, McDonald *et al.* 2006, Powell and Davies 2012, Rowley and Waring 2011). Although professionals' and patients' views may often coincide, our findings suggest that obtaining patients views requires them to have time and space for reflection. Unpacking accounts of preferences concerning GP consultations and their relationship to safety is a complex task which takes time. Our study also highlights the importance of processes to facilitate shared understandings. In the absence of such mechanisms, patients are likely to continue to use the strategies we describe, which may avoid harm, but are likely to expose them to risk at the same time.

Acknowledgements

We thank all our participants for giving their time and sharing their experiences and views for this study. We also wish to thank anonymous references for their very helpful comments and suggestions on previous versions of this chapter.

This research was funded by the National Institute of Health Research School for Primary Care, London, UK, [NIHR School for Primary Care Research (NSPCR) project number 140 UKCRN ID 13694]. The views expressed are those of the authors and not necessarily those of the NHS, the NIHR or the Department of Health.

References

Amalberti, R., Benhamou, D., Auroy, Y. and Degos, L. (2011) Adverse events in medicine: Easy to count, complicated to understand, and complex to prevent, *Journal of Biomedical Informatics*, 44, 3, 390–4.

Brown, P. (2008) Trust in the new NHS: instrumental vs. communicative action, *Sociology of Health and Illness*, 30, 3, 349–60.

Burgess, C., Cowie, L. and Gulliford, M. (2012) Patients' perceptions of error in long-term illness care: qualitative study, *Journal of Health Services Research and Policy*, 17, 3, 181–7.

Chew-Graham, C.A., Hunter, C., Langer, S., Stenhoft, A., *et al.* (2013) How QOF is shaping primary care review consultations: a longitudinal qualitative study, *BMC Family Practice*, 14, 103.

Corbin, J. and Strauss, A. (eds.) (2008) *Basics of Qualitative Research: Techniques and Procedures for Developing Grounded Theory*. Thousand Oaks, CA: Sage.

Coyle, J. (1999) Exploring the meaning of 'dissatisfaction' with health care: the importance of 'personal identity threat', *Sociology of Health & Illness*, 21, 1, 95–123.

Cunliffe, A. and Coupland, C. (2012) From her to villain to hero: Making experience sensible through embodied narrative sensemaking, *Human Relations*, 65, 1, 63–88.

Currie, G., Humpreys, M., Waring, J. and Rowley, E. (2009) Narratives of professional regulation and patient safety: the case of medical devices in anaesthetics, *Health, Risk and Society*, 11, 2, 117–35.

Doherty, C. and Saunders, M.N.K. (2013) Elective surgical patients' narratives of hospitalization: the co-construction of safety, *Social Science & Medicine*, 98, 1, 29–36.

Elder, N.C., Jacobson, C.J., Zink, T. and Hasse, L. (2005) How experiencing preventable medical problems changed patients' interactions with primary health care, *Annals of Family Medicine*, 3, 6, 537–44.

Fotaki, M. (2014) Can consumer choice replace trust in the National Health Service in England? Towards developing an affective psychosocial conception of trust in health care, *Sociology of Health & Illness*, 36, 8, 1276–94.

Giddens, A. (1990) *The Consequences of Modernity*, Bristol: Polity.

Hernan, A.L., Walker, C., Fuller, J., Johnson, J.K., *et al.* (2014) Patients' and carers' perceptions of safety in rural general practice, *Medical Journal of Australia*, 201, (Suppl 3), S60–3.

Hill, A. and Freeman, G. (2011) *Promoting continuity of care in general practice, RCGP Policy Paper, March.* London: The Royal College of General Practitioners.

Hor, S.Y., Iedema, R., Williams, K., White, L., *et al.* (2010) Multiple accountabilities in incident reporting and management, *Qualitative Health Research*, 20, 8, 1091–100.

Hor, S.Y., Godbold, N., Collier, A. and Iedema, R. (2013) Finding the patient in patient safety, *Health*, 17, 6, 567–83.

Horlick-Jones, T. (2005) On 'risk work': Professional discourse, accountability, and everyday action, *Health, Risk and Society*, 7, 3, 293–307.

Hrisos, S. and Thomson, R. (2013) Seeing it from both sides: do approaches to involving patients in improving their safety risk damaging the trust between patients and healthcare professionals? An Interview Study, *PLOS ONE*, 8, 11, e80759.

Iedema, R., Jorm, C., Braithwaite, J., Trevaglia, J., *et al.* (2006) A root cause analysis of clinical error: Confronting the disjunction between formal rules and situated clinical activity, *Social Science & Medicine*, 63, 5, 1201–12.

Kuzel, A.J., Woolf, S.H., Gilchrist, V.J., Engel, J.D., *et al.* (2004) Patient reports of preventable problems and harms in primary health care, *Annals of Family Medicine* 2, 4, 333–40.

McDonald, R., Waring, J. and Harrison, S. (2006) Rules, safety and the narrativisation of identity: a hospital operating theatre case study, *Sociology of Health & Illness*, 28, 2, 178–202.

McDonald, R., Cheraghi-Sohi, S., Bayes, S., Morriss, R., *et al.* (2013) Competing and coexisting logics in the changing field of English general medical practice, *Social Science & Medicine*, 93, 47–54.

Mesman, J. (2009) The geography of patient safety: a topical analysis of sterility, *Social Science & Medicine*, 69, 12, 1705–12.

Nettleton, S., Burrows, R. and Watt, I. (2008) Regulating medical bodies? The consequences of the modernisation of the NHS and the disembodiment of clinical knowledge, *Sociology of Health & Illness*, 30, 3, 333–48.

Powell, A.E. and Davies, H.T. (2012) The struggle to improve patient care in the face of professional boundaries, *Social Science & Medicine*, 75, 5, 807–14.

Rhodes, P., Sanders, C. and Campbell, S. (2014) Relationship continuity: when and why do primary care patients think it is safer? *British Journal of General Practice*, 64, 629, e758–64.

Rhodes, P., Campbell, S. and Sanders, C. (2015) Trust, temporality and systems: how do patients understand patient safety in primary care? A qualitative study, *Health Expectations*, doi:10.111/hex.12342.

Rowley, E. and Waring, J. (eds.). (2011) *A socio-cultural perspective on patient safety*. Farnham, Surrey: Ashgate Publishing.

Scobie, A. (2011) Self-reported medical, medication and laboratory error in eight countries: risk factors for chronically ill adults, *International Journal for Quality in Health Care*, 23, 2, 182–6.

Smith, L.K., Pope, C. and Botha, J.L. (2005) Patients' help-seeking experiences and delay in cancer presentation: a qualitative synthesis, *The Lancet*, 366, 9488, 825–31.

Swinglehurst, D., Greenhalgh, T., Russell, J. and Myall, M. (2011) Receptionist input to quality and safety in repeat prescribing in UK general practice: ethnographic case study, *BMJ*, 343, d6788.

Vincent, C., Burnett, S. and Carthey, J. (2013) *The measurement and monitoring of safety, Spotlight Report April*. London: Health Foundation.

Waring, J. (2009) Constructing and reconstructing narratives of patient safety, *Social Science and Medicine*, 69, 12, 1722–31.

Weick, K. (1995) *Sensemaking in Organizations*. Thousand Oaks, CA: Sage.

Weick, K. (2012) Organized Sensemaking: a commentary on processes of interpretive work, *Human Relations*, 65, 1, 141–53.

Weick, K., Sutcliffe, K. and Obstfeld, D. (2005) Organizing and the process of sensemaking, *Organization Science*, 16, 4, 409–21.

World Health Organisation. (2009) *More than words. Conceptual framework for the international classification for patient safety*. Version 1.1. Final Technical report. Geneva: WHO

Yeung, K. and Dixon-Woods, M. (2010) Design-based regulation and patient safety: a regulatory studies perspective, *Social Science & Medicine*, 71, 3, 502–9.

7

Chains of (dis)trust: exploring the underpinnings of knowledge-sharing and quality care across mental health services

Patrick R. Brown and Michael W. Calnan

Introduction

Effective learning organisations facilitate the refinement and efficient circulation of knowledge of high quality practices, while identifying and applying lessons from contexts or incidents where adverse consequences are experienced (Department of Health [DoH] 2000, Sheaff and Pilgrim 2006, Walshe 2003). Numerous policy interventions in the English National Health Service, within which the current study was conducted, have sought to enhance quality and safety (e.g., DoH 1997, 2005, 2008), often focusing on organisational communication and knowledge management, but with mixed outcomes (Alaszewski 2005, Dixon-Woods *et al.* 2014, Sheaff and Pilgrim 2006, Waring 2005).

Informal organisational cultures are fundamental to quality and safety practices in terms of information sharing (Waring and Bishop 2010) and the impact of quality governance (Brown 2011, Waring 2007). Ormrod (2003), however, indicates the danger that the concept of culture may become a vague residual epithet, used by policymakers and analysts to categorise organisational phenomena lying beyond their control and comprehension. In this study we explore very specific features of organisational culture – that of interwoven relations of (dis)trust across organisations – which bear fundamentally on the communicative and learning functioning of local healthcare services. Far from capturing all of organisational 'culture', our analysis nevertheless identifies salient processes that help explain important 'patterns of relationships and meaning' (Ormrod 2003: 230) across organisations and beyond.

Our analysis functions in between, thus connecting, the 'facework' of (dis)trusting interpersonal interactions and broader cultural tendencies towards (dis)trust, communication and learning (Brown and Calnan 2012, Calnan and Rowe 2008, Davies and Mannion 2000, Sheaff and Pilgrim 2006). Such connections, alongside the theorising of trust as a 'meso-level concept' (Rousseau *et al.* 1998: 394), have been neglected, especially in studies of health policy and sociology (Gilson *et al.* 2005) but also in organisational studies. Across these fields, a dualism exists between more sui generis analyses of dyadic relations, largely independent of context or employing poorly operationalised understandings of how context is influential (Cook *et al.* 2004: 66), and studies of more diffuse networks of actors and organisational systems which lack specific mechanisms for explaining shifts towards (dis)trust (Tan and Lim 2009).

The Sociology of Healthcare Safety and Quality, First Edition. Edited by Davina Allen, Jeffrey Braithwaite, Jane Sandall and Justin Waring. Chapters © 2016 The Authors. Book Compilation © 2016 Foundation for the Sociology of Health & Illness/Blackwell Publishing Ltd.

Trust has been seen as fundamental for quality healthcare provision and outcomes in many national and local healthcare contexts (Brownlie 2008, Calnan and Rowe 2008, Dibben and Lean 2003, Mechanic and Meyer 2000, Sheaff and Pilgrim 2006), enabling action, cooperation and knowledge-sharing where these are otherwise problematic (Adler 2001). Existing empirical research indicates possible linkages between different relationships (see especially Gilson *et al.* 2005): whereby manager-professional trust shapes 'workplace trust' and cooperation between professionals; and where the resulting inter-professional trust impacts on trust building activities between clinicians and patients which, in turn, shapes quality of care (Gilson *et al.* 2005). More broadly, quasi-external governance arrangements, based on policy-makers' apparent mistrust of doctors, may lead to the development of 'structures, policies and processes' (Cook *et al.* 2004, Gillespie and Dietz 2009), which support and/or stifle the communicative cultures through which trust and organisational learning are generated (Adler 2001, Sheaff and Pilgrim 2006).

The impact of broader policy-organisational structures and related managerial priorities may be especially palpable in the English NHS mental healthcare service – especially in services for patients diagnosed with psychosis – where risk management has become a defining policy goal and consequent organisational preoccupation (Langan 2010) and where media depictions of services have emphasised their poor quality (Burns and Priebe 1999). Policy frameworks may therefore not only affect the structuring of workplace interactions (Gilson *et al.* 2005) but impact more directly on trust by influencing how the competency and interests of professionals and managers are considered, respectively, by service users and professionals (Calnan and Rowe 2008, Giddens 1990, Warner 2006).

Theoretical framework: trust chains

Theoretical understandings of the interlinking of different trust relationships across healthcare settings remain nascent and largely descriptive (Gilson *et al.* 2005). Analyses can be thickened through phenomenological insights, by recognising the extent to which interactions are characterised by inferential interpretations of proximal or more distant others (Schutz 1972), in light of more explicit or implicit understandings of the policy priorities, rules and organisational dynamics of wider 'abstract systems' (Giddens 1990: 122, see also Acemoglu and Wolitzky 2012, Gillespie and Dietz 2009, Zimmerman 1971).

The working definition of trust applied in this chapter follows Möllering (2005, 2006), among others. Trust emerges through interpretations and assumptions of compatible agendas or interests, alongside the bracketing off of doubts, which enable positive expectations and thus cooperation regarding a future outcome, amid circumstances characterised by vulnerability and uncertainty. The trustee must also be inferred as sufficiently capable of bringing about positive outcomes (Das and Teng 2001) – hence interests and competencies are two fundamental pillars of trust (Calnan and Rowe 2008).

The salience of inferred interests for trusting relations

Contributing to organisational studies of learning and effectiveness within knowledge intensive environments, Adler (2001) denotes three bases of trust: familiarity, calculation of the interests of others, and awareness of binding norms and values. A recognition of these bases can usefully inform the conceptualisation of how interactions and priorities in one relationship influence trust-building and thus information-sharing activities elsewhere. Changes to trust (or its alternatives, where trust is limited) in one relationship (e.g., between managers and healthcare professionals) impact upon communicative interactions across other relationships (e.g., between healthcare professionals), changing the levels of familiarity and interpretations of converging or diverging interests. Similarly, when shared norms and values are interpreted as becoming more or less binding, then (dis)trust within these other relations is likely to be affected as a result.

Drawing on phenomenology and ethnomethodology, Möllering (2006: 57) indicates the complementarity of familiarity, calculated interests, and compatible norms and values when he argues that interpersonal trust is not so much dependent on the individual trustee herself as on the existence of certain social norms and values in which this trustee's actions are embedded. Such constraining normative structures render a trustee's future actions more 'predictable' (Möllering 2005: 292), in contrast to what we might call loose cannons. Greater levels of familiarity mean the truster presumes that she has a deeper understanding of the social norms and values (institutions) which bear upon the trustee and her degree of embeddedness within these (Zimmerman 1971). This leads the truster to consider herself as being capable of making a more reliable calculation of the trustee's interests and likely behaviour – facilitating (dis)trust.

Emphasising the salience of normative contexts for trust (Möllering 2005) draws our attention to two fundamental environmental features of modern bureaucratic healthcare: *instrumental* bureaucratic pressures towards rendering healthcare work consistent, verifiable and evidence-based, which may potentially complement or impinge upon more *communicative,* person-centred processes focused upon shared understandings and consensus-building (Habermas 1987). Where a manager or professional trustee (for example) is interpreted by a potential truster as being insufficiently embedded within the instrumental or communicative logics, or rather, too deeply embedded in the one and not in the other, then trust becomes problematic (Brown 2008). Policy changes at healthcare system and local organisation levels may also be interpreted as indicating a shift in the structuring of individual interests towards instrumental/ strategic or communicative logics, accordingly assisting or undermining trust.

Interests, vulnerabilities and uncertainties as lynchpins in (dis)trust chains

Interests and norms are central in explaining possibilities for trust but are also decisively shaped by contexts in which trusting occurs (Dirks and Ferrin 2001) and by the bureaucratic checking that takes place in organisations in the relative absence of trust (Davies and Mannion 2000). In any one relationship changing forms of trusting or checking are likely to influence the day-to-day behaviour and interactions of the actors involved (Calnan and Rowe 2008). These modifications, in turn, may have important implications for the (interpreted) interests of these actors and the continuing compatibility – or incompatibility – of their interests with those of other actors within other relationships.

The position of various actors, particularly (manager-)professionals, as both trustees (within one relationship) *and* trusters (within other relationships) is crucial to the generation of chains of (dis)trust across organisations, as are their experiences of, and responses to, vulnerability amid uncertainty (as summarised in Figure 1).

Vulnerability and uncertainty make trust necessary (Möllering 2006), are transformed through trust – where trust offers a solution to vulnerability while the actor also becomes more vulnerable when trusting – and exist in heightened levels when trust is lacking. An actor's solution to this changing vulnerability amid uncertainty will be new forms of more communicative and/or instrumental action – such as voicing and sharing concerns with other actors (communicative) or resorting to checking, evasive or defensive practice (instrumental/ strategic) – as oriented by whether she feels trusted or not, alongside the norms and envisaged possibilities of her culture and identity and the demands imposed on her within social contexts (Habermas 1987). More communicative action may heighten familiarity and

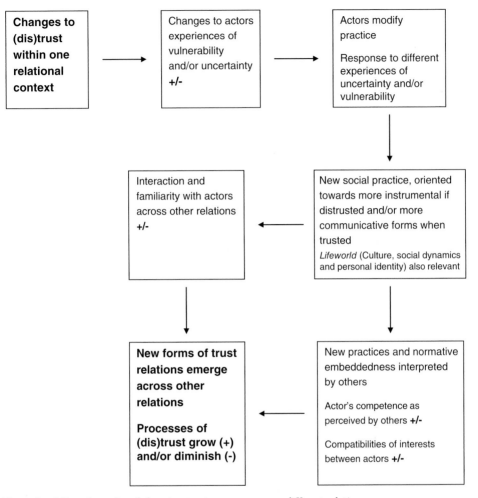

Figure 1   *Micro-dynamics of changing trust processes across different relations*

knowledge-sharing which, as argued earlier, is relevant to trusters' presumed knowledge of the interests of trustees (Adler 2001). More strategic and bureaucratic behaviour, alternatively, may impinge detrimentally upon relations and hinder familiarity, as well as stifle learning.

That these key concepts of interests, vulnerability and uncertainty are each influential upon, and outcomes of, (dis)trust make them vital lynchpins in explaining chains of (dis)trust and thus the broader virtuous and vicious 'cycles' which Gilson *et al.* (2005: 1427) tentatively point towards and which have been observed in organisational studies (Bevan and Hood 2006, Ostrom 2005).

Effective and detailed analyses of the micro-level mechanisms through which cultures of trust or distrust are propagated are vital to sociological studies of quality and safety due to the multifarious ways in which trusting relations underpin quality healthcare practices both directly, as a component of quality patient experiences (Calnan and Rowe 2008), and indirectly by facilitating patients' sharing of information (illuminating needs and appropriate care) (Brown and Calnan 2013) the flow of knowledge within healthcare organisations (Sheaff and Pilgrim 2006) and the development of other capabilities to meet needs effectively and efficiently. The analysis below explores the mechanisms of such linkages between different trust relationships and their interwovenness with interpersonal communication, organisational learning and quality care.

Methods

Approach and design
Conceptualising trust as a process involving the sense-making experiences of actors and the way these are drawn upon when inferring knowledge about actors, groups and organisations (Gillespie and Dietz 2009) suggested the utility of a phenomenological approach, which informed our research design, interviews and data analysis. The taken-for-grantedness (Schutz 1972) in which trust processes are embedded renders them difficult to research, hence Bijlsma-Frankema and Klein-Woolthuis (2005) suggest the utility of studying trust in destabilised contexts. The experiences of psychosis service users, professionals and managers all involve unusually heightened uncertainty and vulnerability. These mental health services thus constituted low trust environments (Pilgrim *et al.* 2011), yet researching three contrasting services granted some variation in trust dynamics. These services were purposively selected in order to explore the varying extent, nature and relevance of (dis)trust across different team and care dynamics. Trust relations and their effects were explored across these three sub-cases – early intervention and assertive outreach services, alongside a standard community mental health team, all in one NHS Trust (local health authority) in southern England – through semi-structured interviews with service users, healthcare professionals and managers (*N* = 21). Interviews with a carer and area chaplain were used to further deepen understandings.

Sampling and participants
Table 1 provides an overview of the professional and manager participants per service. Some of the professionals had considerable experience although this varied (mean = 16.1 years working in mental health services, SD = 10.6). Recruiting service users (eight users and one carer targeted per service) proved much more problematic. Inclusion criteria were service users aged 18 and over, while only those who were experiencing a more acute phase of their illness were excluded. Despite a number of different recruitment strategies and distributing invitation letters to 158 participants, only eight service users (see Table 1) were interviewed.

The service user participants nevertheless reflected a diverse range of backgrounds and experiences (mean duration of contact with services = 15.9 years; SD = 12.4), spanning sex (four men, four women), age range (from 25 to 67), education levels (from leaving school at

Table 1   *Participants' characteristics (n)*

Type of service	Service users	Healthcare professionals	Service managers
Early intervention	2	4 (consultant, assistant psychologist, social worker, community psychiatric nurse (CPN)	1
Assertive outreach	1	3 (consultant, social worker, CPN).	1
Standard community	5	3 (consultant, social worker, CPN).	1

16 to postgraduate study and increments in between) and economic activity (out-of-work, voluntary work, paid-part-time work, retired). Two had less than 2 years' contact with services while the remainder had at least 10 years' experience.

The very low response and sample bias make it likely that the problems of trust our data indicate may in fact be much more profound, especially among certain ethnic minority groups who were absent from our sample (Appleby 2008). This latter limitation, alongside broader recruitment problems, may reflect the vulnerability of the target population, the practical and ethical difficulties associated with this (Smith 2008) and the limited possibilities to adopt a more flexible recruitment strategy due to NHS bureaucracy research governance. When our initial attempts at recruiting users via services were unsuccessful, our adjustments to our access protocols took several months to be endorsed, which, combined with the deadlines of the research funder, limited our possibilities for experimenting with and pursuing different tactics. Our distance from potential user-participants in the recruitment process, having to contact participants by letters that were mailed out by the services, means that we can only speculate on the reasons for our low response rate. One lesson that emerged from these experiences was the desirability of contacting service users through users' networks (both organised and informal) rather than through the NHS services themselves. These alternatives would limit the dependence of the researchers on NHS research governance and, more importantly, limit the possible contamination of the research by low-trust organisations.

Data collection

Interviews with staff typically lasted 30 minutes to one hour and were thematic in format, addressing issues of working with and relating to service users, how positive outcomes were pursued, and the challenges of the job. As with all the interviews, although trust was the central focus of the research, direct questions about the concept were placed later on in the interviews in order to examine the relevance of trust as it emerged 'naturally' within the participants' accounts. Later questions then probed different (dis)trust relations and the nature, influence and (ir)relevance of trust.

Service user and carer interviews followed a longer (50 mins to 1 hour 45 mins), more narrative format, accessing the broader contextual experiences that influenced trust and considering the development of trust or distrust as processes that changed over time in their depth and nature (Möllering 2006). Emerging themes were revisited towards the end of the interview, along with key questions that had not emerged initially in the narratives. The study was given local NHS ethics committee and research governance approval. Interviews took place throughout 2010.

Method of analysis

The interview recordings were transcribed, read multiple times and coded (in NVivo). Basic coding was carried out after each interview in order for emergent themes to inform later interviews. Coding involved open, axial and selective stages (Neuman 1997) by which 'open' refers to the identification of a broad range of potentially relevant factors, partially sensitised by the phenomenological approach outlined above, which directed attention to the apparent assumptions and meaning constructions of the participants (Smith and Osborn 2003). Axial coding used the ongoing (re)delineation and (re)connection of events and concepts into a coherent framework, highlighting recurring and salient processes and linkages.

These more developed understandings were then further refined and nuanced through selective application across individual accounts and events, paying particular attention to deviant cases and the implications of these for overall interpretations. The triangulation of managerial, professional and user insights into different relationships (Cook *et al.* 2004), especially in light of differing dynamics in each of the service sub-cases, aimed to augment internal validity in developing theoretical insights out of a case-study approach (Eisenhardt 1989). To this end we paid much attention to the various participants' narratives about their different relationships with specific individuals and their more general views within the organisational context, as these had developed over time, as well as considering their sense-making of local service contexts and the NHS more generally. Double-coding and critical discussions around the coding process between the researchers and other academic and clinical colleagues assisted the interpretive rigour of the analysis.

Findings

The data presented below illustrate the predominant themes emerging within the analysis, while also acknowledging differences and nuances between sub-cases (services). We particularly focus upon various antecedents and consequences of trust in identifying chains of (dis) trust as these stretched from policymakers to service users.

Quality and performance governance impacting on workplace trust

Uncertainty was a pervasive theme across participants' narratives, and was considered by senior professionals as defining their work (diagnosis, risk assessment and prescribing).

Consultant psychiatrist 2: psychiatry is all about uncertainty

NHS quality governance, not least in mental healthcare, has sought to reduce uncertainty by standardising clinical practice, modifying the formats of inter-professional work and supervision, instituting automatic inquiries into fatalities, together with the routinised coordination of care provision and setting up performance targets and monitoring (among various other reforms). Policymakers and (accordingly) senior managers have thus attempted to 'control' various practices and scrutinise outcomes, attempting to reduce services' vulnerability to efficiency pressures and, perhaps above all, to the political and media criticism associated with high-profile homicides or suicides committed by mental health service users (Pilgrim and Ramon 2009).

Squeezed between such policy (and societal) demands for calculability on the one hand and intractable uncertainty on the other, middle managers and senior clinicians interpreted services as marked by pressure. Quasi-external governance, emphasising checking rather than trust (imposed by policy-makers via senior managers), accordingly created experiences of vulnerability:

Service manager 1: I think there's an awful lot of pressure around ... particularly ... how the services are managed centrally and commissioned. But there is a greater requirement ... people talk about performance targets and we're becoming very orientated towards that [...] but that creates a pressure in itself.[1]

The reorientation of work to satisfy quality and performance pressures was referred to by this manager above as translating into pressure further down the organisation. This was described as a pervasive and growing feature of work by many professionals:

Consultant psychiatrist 2: Increasing pressure all the time. It's not only the reputation [of the organisation amid media scrutiny of adverse incidents], it's about lots of things:

it's government targets, it's the organisational targets, it's what they call 'serious untoward incidents'. All of this happens all the time, and it's becoming even more ...

When asked how their role had changed, middle managers referred to their expanding responsibilities to oversee various features emphasised within new policies, not least productivity, professional performance and quality development:

> Service manager 2: We're expected much more now to manage things like annual leave and sickness and training. And all those things didn't seem to be at the forefront maybe 10, 15 years ago but now ... managing your team effectively with the resources, how we deliver the service, it's very much in the forefront.

Implementing and policing the performance and quality directives designed by senior counterparts were described by middle managers as shaping their relationships with professionals. Different participants believed that growing bureaucracy was both a cause and an effect of the deteriorating trust relations and familiarity between professionals and managers:

> Consultant psychologist 1: I think there's a bigger distance between senior clinicians and managers than there used to be. So that's changed. Clinicians, I think, are less involved in big decisions; which can be problematic. But ... I think that's a question of trust. I think maybe we lost the trust of [senior] managers somewhere along the line, by thinking we knew it all.

This erosion of trusting relations can partly be understood through the working definition introduced earlier – growing incompatibilities between the interests of senior managers and those of professionals:

> Community psychiatric nurse 4: We can't trust the high up managers ... . We can't trust them because they have a different agenda and they're not telling us everything, and I know that sounds like a conspiracy theory but they're not ... And ... well, everybody's [concerned] about number crunching.

Middle managers, with whom professionals were more familiar, were referred to much less frequently as being distrusted. Instead, the bureaucratic demands these latter managers implemented were often perceived as a consequence of more senior directorates:

> Social worker 1: The managers higher up ... they've probably got aims and outcomes that they've got to prove. So, in regards to kind of doing paperwork, keeping up contacts and doing any audit things – a lot of that is affected and we probably all find that our paperwork is very time consuming and [...] most of us feel quite frustrated that we can't be doing more things [with service users].

Pressure towards effectiveness, imposed by senior managers – who were also seen as being constrained by policy frameworks – and implemented by middle managers manifested itself as stress for many professionals working amid uncertainty. When asked what was challenging about the job, social worker 2 recounted:

> Social worker 2: Every day, just facing different issues on a day to day basis and that's really quite stressful ... paperwork and keeping up to date with that as well, that's

difficult in itself, making sure everything's on the computer and you've got it all up to date. But it's just being faced with different scenarios every day, and not knowing whether you've done the right thing or not by that client.

One important and more common narrative was on the impact of such stress via sickness absences or retention problems:

Social worker 2: We get stressed and so staff go off sick, so obviously, you need to look after someone's caseload as well.
Consultant psychiatrist 2: Well, that's why everybody's understaffed … ['juggling' financial pressures and pressure over managing risk].
Interviewer: Really?
Consultant psychiatrist 2: That's why staff opt out all the time. And even if they don't leave the whole mental health services, they just move from one place to the other because they're just restless, because of the anxiety … I mean, I find myself quite fortunate because I'm a person who can deal with that [stress] … but I'm struggling with the fact that the rest of the team I work with are not, and they are always under stress of people leaving and vacancies and so on.

Heterogeneous accounts of 'vulnerability' and resilience were thus apparent. The accounts of senior staff suggested they were more insulated from stress, partly due to their distance from specific cases and their greater decision-making discretion and autonomy (Wainwright and Calnan 2002). Among lower level professionals, however, levels of absence due to sickness were commonly referred to as a serious issue in two of the three services. This difference was also reflected in the form of narratives (as apparent above). Whereas senior manager-professionals described stress in a more distanced, third-person manner, more junior professionals referred to their own direct experiences in the first person.

Sickness absence resulting from work stress was referred to as a manifestation of vulnerability, resulting from the (instrumental) scrutiny and checking on professionals within management frameworks, which in turn were a response to policy-rooted vulnerabilities noted earlier, alongside the uncertainty of everyday work. Absences were also interpreted as creating difficulties in building effective inter-professional relations and providing quality care:

Manager 1: If someone is sick a lot or off a lot and not contributing to the team in those types of things, and then it starts to feel a little bit uneasy and people start to have splitting and those types of things. They can't trust that the person is gonna be there all the time, meetings get cancelled, or CPAs [care coordination meetings] get cancelled, and that's when the trust starts to unbalance and shift the team around; things like that, commitment to work; that one that comes up here quite a lot.

Sickness absences therefore represented one rather palpable linkage through which the vulnerability of professionals amidst governance and management structures impacted on inter-professional trust, knowledge-sharing opportunities and effectiveness.

Inter-professional relations: shaping productivity and learning

Obstacles to trust were frequently apparent within participant narratives, yet more positive accounts of trust were not uncommon. One manager of a service which was newer and seemingly better resourced than the others explained she had high trust in her colleagues, emphasising a need to trust for the sake of efficiency:

> Service manager 3: I have to trust people … that they're doing what they're employed to do … . I can't go around looking at everybody's caseloads and making sure that there's a care plan in there, there's a risk assessment in there, that they've printed out their contact records. I have to … you know, delegate.

Relying on trust could, in turn, create efficiencies within the team due to the lack of checking (see later in this section). Yet even in this team, where the service manager described trusting competent colleagues, more overarching governance structures ('the whole system') impinged on professional time, shaping interests and practices, as reported by this senior professional:

> Consultant psychologist 1: It's related to the trustworthiness or untrustworthiness of the whole system, because [my] colleagues' record-keeping is often defensive, in my view. So they write reams and reams and reams of contact details just in case they … if they're ever called to account.

Despite the service manager's aims, accountability pressures imposed via senior management were nevertheless experienced by professionals as rendering them vulnerable, which they described mitigating through bureaucratic-instrumental practice. Vulnerabilities, such as those relating to clinical uncertainty, could also be attended to via more communicative-relational means, such as supervision and support from fellow professionals:

> Consultant psychologist 1: [There is] that wish to find certainty about diagnosis or prediction and prognosis – to know exactly when someone's going to hurt themselves or someone else – and trying to live with the fact that you can't predict those things with anything like the degree of certainty that we'd want. So we use supervision; especially group supervision is often taken up with that.

As with spending time with service users (see next section), more communicative-relational approaches such as supervision (formal and informal) were a common way in which professionals and managers referred to dealing with vulnerability amidst uncertainty. For more junior professionals in the team this was a vital means of learning and being supported. Supervision was understood as combining communicative activity (sharing experiences and understandings) with instrumental development (teaching and facilitating better or safer outcomes):

> Assistant psychologist: I think there's times when I've thought 'Oh, I've really not handled something very well' … I've kind of gone in the next day and gone 'that was just awful' and … . So I think that's quite often that … people offload a bit … Yeah, I think that's quite helpful and yes, that is a trusting thing isn't it – to be able to do that.

Similarly, for senior professionals and managers, supervision was described as a way of providing communicative support as well as ensuring key instrumental functions were fulfilled. As is apparent from the excerpts above and below, reciprocal trust was said to be vital to effective supervision:

> Consultant psychiatrist 3: The trust relationship is very important … you rely on them and you see difficult cases with them and support them in difficult cases – and they

support you. And we are, with the 'new ways of working', for the psychiatrists we have to have … more of an advisory role.

Here the psychiatrist's development of trusting relationship is interpreted within the limits imposed by the policy framework (DoH 2005) in which he worked. This reduced his hands-on role with service users and therefore could render interactions with and trust in colleagues more necessary, as a way of coping with this more advisory function. More senior participants thus also referred to 'relying' upon or being supported by their junior colleagues amidst trust relations, as well as being depended upon themselves. Trust relations within governance frameworks which rendered senior practitioners vulnerable were therefore not as neatly vertical as one might assume.

Yet, as beneficial as interactive learning and support could be, excessive supervision sessions and other meetings were also referred to as potentially eroding time with service users:

Social worker 3: There's lots of supervision – you've already picked up on that?! … I'd say client time is probably only a third but the reason for that is because of travel, meetings and paperwork.

Supervision and group meetings were interpreted as sometimes being more concerned with checking on professionals' work (surveillance) than with constructive learning and support. In some cases these experiences of checking were related to the broader bureaucratising tendencies of the NHS. Instrumental-strategic action could in this way function 'parasitically' through ostensibly communicative processes (Habermas 1987: 187, Weiss 1979). Distinctions between trust and checking (Adler 2001, Davies and Mannion 2000) are important here in distinguishing between aspects of supervision which, facilitated by trust, were described as enabling the sharing of useful knowledge and mutual learning and those that were held to serve the function of verification and auditing while consuming time.

Time has been found to play a vital role in trust relations (Dibben and Lean 2003). It emerged within the interview narratives as one further fundamental element which – as both an antecedent and product of trust – was described as relevant in interlinkages between trust relations. Too many formal meetings and too much paperwork was seen as reducing the availability and flexibility of professionals. This was interpreted as impacting profoundly upon their relations with service users (see next section) but was also described as influencing their relations with colleagues. In one service which had comparatively few meetings, this more junior professional indicated the accessibility and consequent support of his colleagues:

Social worker 2: Because, you know, I think any problem, any issues – there's always someone around that you can speak to and they will take that time out to, kind of, give you advice and, you know, kind of tell you whether you're doing the right thing by that, or give you advice on how maybe to approach situations.

However the availability of this support and supervision, and the trust that was seen earlier as underpinning it, was described by the same professional as being under threat:

Social worker 2: You know … [trust] depends on various factors, how much pressure you are under, how much time you have got … . I mean in terms of … relationship with … clients, to colleagues, you know, to the management, everything! … Now we're getting more pressure so obviously, you know, lack of staff and more cases …

Resource issues, sickness absences, related pressures to take on larger case-loads, alongside governance pressures (as discussed earlier) were referred to as combining to consume time. In contrast, in the service where the manager expressed a particular keenness to trust colleagues (see the start of this section), professionals understood trusting relations in the team and management as enhancing productivity and commitment:

> Assistant psychologist: … people give more hours than they should really … people feel almost that because we're trusted it … it's almost reciprocal then, you know – 'well, I won't put that half an hour down', you know, 'that's fine'. So actually I think it's probably a lot, lot more productive … and you don't have people spending two hours moaning about the management [as experienced in a previous workplace] because there's not anything to moan about. So, yeah, I think that works really, really well and hopefully it will stay like that.

Professional and service user relations: the importance and hindrance of interaction-time, competence and care

The preceding quotation shows how professionals' interests and practices could be potently shaped by workplace trust relations involving middle management (Gilson *et al.* 2005). Conversely, earlier in the preceding section, productivity and quality decision-making were interpreted as being impeded when supervision became partially colonised as surveillance, or where bureaucratic monitoring was seen as consuming professional time. Professionals' various relations to governance frameworks, management and colleagues – understood as open, trusting communication, and/or defensiveness and experiences of 'pressure' – were interpreted as impacting significantly on professional practice in the service users' narratives:

> Service user 3: I was introduced to the concept of 'key worker' and the first one was absolutely crap and was off [sick] more than he was there.

Sickness absence, as described earlier, was referred to as a serious problem in a number of participants' accounts, contributing directly and indirectly to particular professionals' relational distance from service users.

Users' narratives included many experiences of limited trust in professionals, although most users described at least one professional whom they had trusted. Trust was referred to, explicitly and implicitly, as developing in various ways but most consistently involved interpretations of instrumental competence and communicative relation-building:

> Service user 7: I had a doctor 10 years ago and I think he spent a lot of time to get to know me and he diagnosed me as having something else and […] It really seemed to hit the nail on the head and what I was feeling and what my thoughts were at the time.

Development of relations over time was thus salient for mutual understanding and awareness of interests (needs). Growing familiarity, rapport and trust were recurrently reported by professionals and service users alike as being integral to effective care relationships:

> Service user 8: It just seemed like she kind of had some care and concern, which I'm not saying the other guy didn't, but it just seemed like time was slower there … You have to trust them enough to tell them … you know, it's stuff that you feel ashamed about

really … But it really felt like she just kind of put me right up the list for that period of time and that it really didn't matter what else was going on.

Sensitive information, disclosed within trusting relations, further enabled appropriate assistance and, correspondingly, quality outcomes. Similar processes were also pertinent for professionals, in feeling able to discuss difficult cases with their colleagues and supervisors, but trust and time were especially vital for service users in overcoming stigma and shame (vulnerability) to disclose their difficulties. Time here was as much a subjective basis of experience and meaning-making (Schutz 1972) as an objective resource; a slower 'cadence' of interaction assisting open communication and quality care.

Such positive experiences were likely to have been impeded by sickness absences or the regular rotation of professionals working with particular users due to retention problems (Cook *et al.* 2004). Professionals similarly underlined the importance of time for relation building, as well as its erosion through various processes:

Social worker 2: I think … rapport then depends on the caseload. […] When I started working with the clients … initially and I may have a good rapport and then … I have currently got something approximating 28/30 cases so I would say the last clients on my list may not be … may not have that [rapport] because I don't have enough time to spend with them. So obviously … external factors affect it anyway and the trust. […] And that's changed a lot …
Interviewer: Why is that?
Social worker 2: Because of the pressure of paperwork; because of the pressure of the nature of the work now.

This significance of time and familiarity thus underscores the value of trusting manager-professional and inter-professional relations in freeing up time to devote to users. Similarly, high levels of commitment, described by the professional quoted at the end of the preceding section as being galvanised by managerial trust, could be seen as underpinning quality care and users' inferences of trust:

Service user 3: She is trained to do the job properly and she understands what the job involves and she knows that at times that she will have to make a commitment which is, you know, outlined in her contract of employment, but sometimes a commitment that goes beyond that in order to make sure that clients are safe and that the paperwork's done. But I didn't say anything about how that impacts on me and what that has meant to me over the time that she's been my key worker […] because it's one thing for her to be all these things but if it doesn't have any value or impact for me then it's … it's not that important. I would say that out of all the people I come into contact [with] bar none – including individuals that are not employed by the NHS – I would trust her the most.

These last few lines emphasised subjective, interpretative experiences of care and trust. However such interpretations of training and commitment were also connected to practices of quality training and informal norms of professional duty.

As noted earlier, knowledge-intensive organisations such as mental health services rely on trust among staff to enable sufficient information sharing in order to drive quality care. The effective application of this knowledge was also understood as bearing upon care outcomes and consequently on users' trust (Das and Teng 2001). Management and accountability frameworks were in various ways described by professionals as inhibiting optimal care decisions:

> Psychiatrist 2: Another thing that I think is very difficult is … how much the politics and the dynamics of the organisation interfere with clinical decisions … that I have to practice defensively at some point. […] So I'm of the opinion that due to this sometimes, in psychiatry in particular, sometimes we do not help patients to improve, and on the contrary … we're creating users of the service because some of the things that we do is reinforcing certain behaviour and a certain pattern of thinking … What we need to do maybe is to work on it to try and … well minimise it but instead … because we have to act on the risk and we have to protect ourselves and protect the service, we reinforce it.

It has been argued that such risk-governance approaches lead to the service user being approached as a risk object rather than a human being (Castel 1991), indicating a further indirect and negative influence of policy frameworks, via management and supervisory relations, upon professional–user relations. More directly, the highly publicised risk-focused logics of recent policies within English mental health services (Pilgrim and Ramon 2009), alongside negative individual experiences at access points (especially of inpatient experiences), coalesced towards one general impression of institutional interests diverging from those of users:

> Service user 7: Well they're not interested in you. They're just … They're just there for the daily routine, you know, to make sure that you do all of the things you're supposed to do, and to them you're just a schizophrenic.

Discussion: from trust chains to vicious and virtuous cycles

Central to the analysis above is the identification of (i) a number of processes which are useful in understanding how trusting or distrusting relationships across healthcare organisations may be impacted by, and in turn impact upon, other relationships; (ii) various ways in which processes shaping knowledge-sharing and quality care provision are interwoven within these chains of (dis)trust. The high levels of uncertainty, vulnerability and fragile trust dynamics that existed in the psychosis service settings were useful in making visible key mechanisms and interdependencies that may have remained more hidden or taken-for-granted in high-trust environments (Bijlsma-Frankema and Klein-Woolthuis 2005). This analysis and theorisation is aimed at advancing medical sociological and health policy understandings, partly drawing upon insights from organisational studies (Currie *et al.* 2012).

Trust chains, in proliferating certain relational-communicative and instrumental-strategic tendencies across organisations, assist in explaining the emergence of broader organisational patterns of (dis)trust and (poor) quality care. Vicious or virtuous cycles of trust help capture important cultural underpinnings of knowledge-sharing, learning and performance (Gilson *et al.* 2005). A meso-level analysis of trust chains was built through micro-linkages or lynchpins, understood through vulnerability, interests, uncertainty and time being both antecedents and products of trust. These four lynchpins may be usefully divided between those – vulnerability and interests – which are of most interest to studies of trust, power and control within organisations, and those – uncertainty or knowledge and time – which are most directly relevant to quality and effectiveness. The central mechanisms and many of

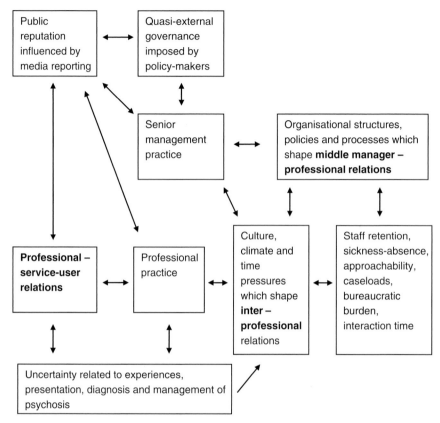

Figure 2   *Salient chains of interwoven relations and components across and beyond mental healthcare organisations*

the concepts in our analytical framework are, through their abstract qualities, likely to be pertinent for many healthcare-organisational contexts. However our findings are in various ways specific to our case study and further or alternative lynch-pins may well be identified across other organisational contexts.

The experiences of individual actors within certain (dis)trusting relations correspondingly enabled or hindered their familiarity and openness with other actors. In our case study, pressures enacted by policymakers and imposed via managers were regularly seen to lead to vulnerability (such as accountability pressures, strenuous workloads and work stress), resulting in instrumental-strategic behaviour (such as taking absence from work, the defensive use of paperwork, defensive clinical practice and reduced interactions with colleagues). Such responses to vulnerability created new forms of uncertainty and vulnerability among managers and professionals (see Figure 2, in which each arrow represents a potential source of vulnerability); for example, through limited communicative time or poor health, which in turn eroded or colonised knowledge-sharing (in the short term), familiarity and relationship formation (in the long term). It follows that new uncertainties and vulnerabilities then tended to emerge for a range of related actors – managers, professionals or users – impacting directly and indirectly on relationships, communication and quality care provision. Again, while uncertainties and vulnerabilities are intrinsic to contexts where trust becomes necessary, these will manifest themselves in many different ways and Figure 2 is by no means comprehensive or exhaustive, even of this one small case study.

Processes around such lynchpins also assist in understanding why vicious circles are far from inevitable. Above we have explored how actors may respond to uncertainty and vulnerability in different ways. The nature of these responses – whether towards more instrumental-strategic formats of behaviour in seeking to defend oneself against uncertainty, or more openly communicative action in seeking to resolve uncertainty through knowledge-sharing, mutual understanding and familiarity – are significant in understanding the generation of vicious circles or, alternatively, virtuous circles of trust. Enduring norms for responding to vulnerability constitute one important basis for understanding the orientation of behaviour (towards more communicative-relational or defensive-bureaucratic), as shaped by organisational, professional and/or socio-biographical contexts. Whether actors felt trusted or not was one key organisational factor.

The linear ordering of the findings sub-sections above implies a 'top-down' chain of trust or, as has often been the case in the data presented here, distrust; one where certain overarching governance frameworks more or less directly shaped working environments and relations which were described as dysfunctional for trust. Importantly, many of these negative pressures resulted from the implementation of quality and performance frameworks.

Yet as was emphasised at the start of the analysis section, certain 'bottom up' tendencies also existed due to the particularly high levels of uncertainty which were described as inherent to the experience of psychosis, both for those with a diagnosis and for those with the responsibility of caring for this vulnerable group of service users. It is the seeming incompatibility between this intractable and heightened uncertainty and the stringent demands for high levels of accountability and monitoring which create such relational tensions for the managers, professionals and users who must interact in the midst of these chains. Chains of (dis)trust may thus stretch right through and beyond an organisation, with the nature of users/patients at one end of the chain, and the policy or legal frameworks at the other, exerting important influences on the relational dynamics in-between.

The conceptual relationships identified here (summarised in Figures 1 and 2) build on existing understandings (Gilson *et al.* 2005) by identifying certain key mechanisms that are fundamental to connections between different trust relations. The conceptual tool of trust chains should not only be applied in a link by link approach, however. Some more complex interlinking across chains is captured in Figure 2. For example, we have noted that although senior managers had little interactive-relational contact with professionals, their policies and the interests inferred from their policy-making nonetheless had an important impact on professional work and sense-making regarding middle management. Senior managers were sometimes typified via policies as 'the organisation', more or less negatively. Policy and management directives could also impact on service users' trust relations with professionals, with the latter actors' typified as being embedded within particular overarching management norms (Möllering 2005). Dynamics of trust chains accordingly function not only through proximal linkages but also via a more distant association or contamination and its resulting impact on actors' interpretative schemes (Schutz 1972).

Phenomenologically grounded conceptualisations of trust chains may thus be unusually powerful at illuminating – though by no means fully capturing – important cultural tendencies that are highly salient to quality and safety practices, if we understand 'organisational culture' as 'patterns of relationships and meaning' (Ormrod 2003: 230). The analytical framework presented here requires further exploration and scrutiny across a range of contexts within and beyond English mental healthcare – including higher-trust organisational and different clinical settings – for further refinement and development. 'Quality' in caring for people with chronic and severe mental health problems, as described by participants in our study, is arguably more of a relational attribute than it is in many other healthcare settings while ambiguity around what quality means is unusually heightened, as are organisational sensitivities towards risk. Nevertheless, all healthcare services rely on successfully refining communicative and instrumental processes, with chains of (dis)trust profoundly influencing cultures of knowledge-sharing, learning and care-giving.

Acknowledgements

The study on which this chapter was based was funded by the UK Economic and Social Research Council grant RES-000–22–3535. The authors are grateful to the service managers, healthcare professionals and above all the service users for their cooperation and involvement in the study. The expert advice of Amanda Scrivener and George Szmukler at different points of the research process was very valuable. The final version of this chapter was importantly enhanced through the quality of the peer reviewers' comments and moreover the suggestions and insights provided by Guido Möllering on an earlier draft of the chapter.

Note

1   An ellipsis is used to indicate a pause or hesitation or in place of recurring expressions such as 'urm', 'kinda', 'like', 'you know' which added little in terms of content and could potentially make the participant more easily identifiable. On a few occasions where participants repeated or restarted a sentence the repetition is omitted and marked with […]. Where one excerpt includes two pieces of transcript which were originally uttered within two distinct sentences this is indicated by a starting a new line.

References

Acemoglu, D. and Wolitzky, A. (2012) Cycles of distrust: an economic model. NBER Working Paper No. 18257. Available at: http://www.nber.org/papers/w18257 (accessed 18 September 2015).
Adler, P. (2001) Market, hierarchy, and trust: the knowledge economy and the future of capitalism, *Organization Science*, 12, 2, 215–34.
Alaszewski, A. (2005) Risk, safety and organisational change in healthcare?, *Health, Risk and Society*, 7, 4, 315–8.
Appleby, L. (2008) Services for ethnic minorities: a question of trust, *Psychiatric Bulletin*, 32, 11, 401–2.
Bevan, G. and Hood, C. (2006) What's measured is what matters: targets and gaming in the English public health care system, *Public Administration*, 84, 3, 517–38.
Bijlsma-Frankema, K. and Klein-Woolthuis, R. (2005) *Trust under Pressure: Empirical Investigations of Trust and Trust Building in Uncertain Circumstances.* Cheltenham: Edward Elgar.
Brown, P. (2008) Trusting in the new NHS: instrumental versus communicative action, *Sociology of Health and Illness*, 30, 3, 349–63.
Brown, P. (2011) The concept of lifeworld as a tool in analysing health-care work: exploring professionals' resistance to governance through subjectivity, norms and experiential knowledge, *Social Theory and Health*, 9, 2, 147–65.
Brown, P. and Calnan, M. (2012) *Trusting on the Edge: Managing Uncertainty and Vulnerability in the Midst of Severe Mental Health Problems.* Bristol: Policy Press.
Brown, P. and Calnan, M. (2013) Trust as a means of bridging the management of risk and the meeting of need: a case study in mental health service provision, *Social Policy & Administration*, 47, 3, 242–61.

Brownlie, J. (2008) Conceptualising trust and health. In Brownlie, J., Greene, A. and Howson, A. (eds) *Researching Trust and Health.* London: Routledge.

Burns, T. and Priebe, S. (1999) Mental healthcare failure in England: myth and reality, *British Journal of Psychiatry,* 174, 3, 191–2.

Calnan, M. and Rowe, R. (2008) *Trust Matters in Healthcare.* Buckingham: Open University Press.

Castel, R. (1991) From dangerousness to risk. In Burchell, G., Gordon, C. and Miller, P. (eds) *The Foucault Effect – Studies in Governmentality.* Hemel Hempstead: Harvester Wheatsheaf.

Cook, K., Kramer, R., Thom, D., Stepanikova, I., *et al.* (2004) Trust and distrust in patient-physician relationships: perceived determinants of high- and low-trust relationships in managed-care settings. In Kramer, R.M. and Cook, K.S. (eds) *Trust and Distrust in Organizations: Dilemmas and Approaches.* New York: Russell Sage Foundation.

Currie, G., Dingwall, R., Kitchener, M. and Waring, J. (2012) Let's dance: organization studies, medical sociology and health policy, *Social Science & Medicine,* 74, 3, 273–80.

Das, T. and Teng, B.-S. (2001) Trust, control and risk in strategic alliances: an integrative framework, *Organization Studies,* 22, 2, 251–83.

Davies, H. and Mannion, R. (2000) Clinical governance: striking a balance between checking and trusting. In Smith, P. (ed) *Reforming Markets in Health Care: an Economic Perspective.* Buckingham: Open University Press.

Department of Health [DoH (1997) *The New NHS: Modern, Dependable.* London: DoH.

DoH (2000) *An Organisation with a Memory: Report of an Expert Group on Learning from Adverse Events in the NHS Chaired by the Chief Medical Officer.* London: The Stationery Office.

DoH (2005) *New Ways of Working for Psychiatrists: Enhancing Effective, Person-Centred Services through New Ways of Working in Multidisciplinary and Multiagency Contexts.* London: DoH.

DoH (2008) *Refocusing the Care Programme Approach: Policy and Positive Practice Guidance.* London: DoH.

Dibben, M. and Lean, M. (2003) Achieving compliance in chronic illness management: illustrations of trust relationships between physicians and nutrition clinic patients, *Health, Risk and Society,* 5, 3, 241–8.

Dirks, K. and Ferrin, D. (2001) The role of trust in organizational settings, *Organization Science,* 12, 4, 450–67.

Dixon-Woods, M., Baker, R., Charles, K., Dawson, J., *et al.* (2014) Culture and behaviour in the English National Health Service: overview of lessons from a large multimethod study, *BMJ: Quality & Safety,* 23, 106–15.

Eisenhardt, K. (1989) Building theories from case study research, *Academy of Managment Review,* 14, 4, 532–50.

Giddens, A. (1990) *The Consequences of Modernity.* Cambridge: Polity.

Gillespie, N. and Dietz, G. (2009) Trust repair after an organization-level failure, *Academy of Management Review,* 34, 1, 127–45.

Gilson, L., Palmer, N. and Schneider, H. (2005) Trust and health worker performance: exploring a conceptual framework using South African evidence, *Social Science & Medicine,* 61, 7, 1418–29.

Habermas, J. (1987) *Theory of Communicative Action. Volume Two: Lifeworld and System: A Critique of Functionalist Reason.* Cambridge: Polity.

Langan, J. (2010) Challenging assumptions about risk factors and the role of screening for violence risk in the field of mental health, *Health, Risk and Society,* 12, 2, 85–100.

Mechanic, D. and Meyer, S. (2000) Concepts of trust among patients with serious illness, *Social Science & Medicine,* 51, 5, 657–68.

Möllering, G. (2005) The trust/control duality: an integrative perspective on positive expectations of others, *International Sociology,* 20, 3, 283–305.

Möllering, G. (2006) *Trust: Reason, Routine, Reflexivity.* Oxford: Elsevier.

Neuman, W. (1997) *Social Research Methods: Qualitative and Quantitative Approaches.* Boston: Allyn and Bacon.

Ormrod, S. (2003) Organisational culture in health service policy and research: 'third-way' political fad or policy development?, *Policy and Politics,* 31, 2, 227–37.

Ostrom, E. (2005) Toward a behavioural theory linking trust, reciprocity and reputation. In Ostrom, E. and Walker, J. (eds) *Trust and Reciprocity: Interdisciplinary Lessons for Experimental Research*. New York: Russell Sage.

Pilgrim, D. and Ramon, S. (2009) English mental health policy under New Labour, *Policy and Politics*, 37, 2, 273–88.

Pilgrim, D., Tomasini, F. and Vassilev, I. (2011) *Examining Trust in Health Care*. Basingstoke: Palgrave Macmillan.

Rousseau, D.M., Sitkin, S.B., Burt, R. and Camerer, C. (1998) Not so different after all: a cross-disciplinary view of trust, *Academy of Management Review*, 23, 3, 1–12.

Schutz, A. (1972) *The Phenomenology of the Social World*. London: Heinemann.

Sheaff, R. and Pilgrim, D. (2006) Can learning organizations survive in the newer NHS, *Implementation Science*, 1, 1–27.

Smith, J. and Osborn, M. (2003) Interpretative phenomenological analysis. In Breakwell G. (ed.) *Doing Social Psychology Research*. Oxford: Blackwell.

Smith, L. (2008) How ethical is ethical research?, *Recruiting marginalized, vulnerable groups into health services research, Journal of Advanced Nursing*, 62, 2, 248–57.

Tan, H.H. and Lim, A. (2009) Trust in co-workers and trust in organizations, *Journal of Psychology*, 143, 1, 45–66.

Wainwright, D. and Calnan, M. (2002) *Work Stress: the Making of a Modern Epidemic*. Buckingham: Open University Press.

Walshe, K. (2003) Understanding and learning from organisational failure, *Quality and Safety in Healthcare*, 12, 2, 81–2.

Waring, J. (2005) Beyond blame: the cultural barriers to medical incident reporting, *Social Science & Medicine*, 60, 9, 1927–35.

Waring, J. (2007) Adaptive regulation or governmentality: patient safety and the changing regulation of medicine, *Sociology of Health & Illness*, 29, 2, 163–79.

Waring, J. and Bishop, S. (2010) Watercooler learning: knowledge sharing at the clinical backstage and its contribution to patient safety, *Journal of Health, Organisation and Management*, 24, 4, 325–42.

Warner, J. (2006) Inquiry reports as active texts and their function in relation to professional practice in mental health, *Health, Risk and Society*, 8, 3, 223–37.

Weiss, C. (1979) The many meanings of research utilization, *Public Administration Review*, 39, 5, 426–31.

Zimmerman, D. (1971) Record keeping and the intake process in a public welfare organization. In Wheeler, S. (ed.) *On Record: Files and Dossiers in American Life*. New York: Russell Sage.

8

Spatio-temporal elements of articulation work in the achievement of repeat prescribing safety in UK general practice

Suzanne Grant, Jessica Mesman and Bruce Guthrie

Introduction

The use of medications that only clinically qualified professionals can prescribe is the most common technical intervention in healthcare. Prescriptions may be one-off to treat a short-lived illness, but three quarters of prescriptions and four-fifths of drug costs in the UK are accounted for by what is referred to in UK general practice as 'repeat prescribing' (Avery 2010). Repeat prescriptions are for chronically-used medications, typically authorised at the last medication review, and issued without a consultation between the patient and prescriber (Audit Commission 1994). Over recent decades, the proportion of items issued as repeat prescriptions has increased in parallel with the expansion in prescribing for long-term conditions in general practice. For example, a recent study by Petty *et al.* (2014) found that at least one repeat medication was prescribed to 43 per cent of the population at any one time, with this increasing to over 75 per cent of the population over 60 years of age.

Repeat prescribing is a high-volume process that involves multiple general practice professionals. UK general practices are typically general practitioner (GP)-owned businesses with 3,000–15,000 patients, which will receive tens or hundreds of requests for repeat prescriptions for hundreds or sometimes thousands of different medications (many patients request multiple medications each time) each day, with a requirement to turn these requests into prescriptions for collection within 24–48 hours. UK general practices make significant use of clinical IT systems, which contain electronic patient records in the processing of repeat prescriptions to record, authorise, and issue repeat prescriptions. Although the signature of a qualified prescriber, usually a doctor, is legally required to issue a prescription, non-clinically trained administrative staff have responsibility for multiple tasks in the process.

Medication errors are a major cause of adverse events, with a recent study (Avery *et al.* 2013) stating that 4.9 per cent of repeat prescriptions contain an error. Given this, the measurement and management of prescribing is an important safety concern for the UK National Health Service (NHS) (Garfield *et al.* 2009, Taylor 1996). Research studies have also identified mild to moderate medication errors as relatively common and caused by a combination of individual factors (e.g. training, fatigue) and organisational factors (e.g. organisational culture, communication). For example, Avery *et al.* (2013) found that only 0.2 per cent of repeat prescription items in their study contained a severe error. While this research has been important for understanding the reasons why errors occur, it does not capture in

---

The Sociology of Healthcare Safety and Quality, First Edition. Edited by Davina Allen, Jeffrey Braithwaite, Jane Sandall and Justin Waring. Chapters © 2016 The Authors. Book Compilation © 2016 Foundation for the Sociology of Health & Illness/Blackwell Publishing Ltd.

detail the socio-cultural complexities of healthcare organisation and delivery, including differences in perceptions and definitions of risk and safety across organisational contexts and professional groups. In order to address these shortcomings, recent research on patient safety and quality improvement has emphasised the importance of organisational context and the complex power dynamics that operate therein on the way that risk is understood and quality and safety achieved (Iedema 2009, Macrae 2014, Rowley and Waring 2011, The Health Foundation 2014).

An important development within this emerging field of research has been the achievement of more nuanced understandings of the relationship between formal structural understandings and expressions of safety and informal everyday practice. In these studies, 'safety' is understood as a continuous enactment of the collective orientation of teams to each other, their resources, their physical environments, and their tasks (Iedema *et al.* 2014). One analytical lens that has been fruitfully applied within the context of secondary and community care has been Strauss's concept of 'articulation work' (Strauss 1985, 1988, 1993, Strauss *et al.* 1997). This concept has been used to examine the nature of collaborative activities between health and community care professionals, and the informal and often 'invisible' knowledge and resources that are necessary to conduct this work (e.g. Allen 2014, Hampson and Junior 2005, Postma *et al.* 2014, Timmermans and Freidin 2007). The concept of articulation work covers both formal routinized work and informal un/planned responses to un/anticipated contingencies (Allen 2014, Star 1991). Within the context of repeat prescribing, this work is dependent on the successful coordination of work between GPs and receptionists.

Receptionists have a central role in general practice work, with one of their key responsibilities being to act as administrative gatekeepers to GPs (Arber and Sawyer 1985, Ward and McMurray 2011). In the literature, the work of receptionists has often been contrasted with other members of the general practice team, in particular that of GPs (Copeman and Van Zwanenberg 1988). The majority of extant research on receptionists has focused on their role at the practice front desk and the extent to which they were understood and valued by patients (Hammond *et al.* 2013, Hewitt *et al.* 2009). Fewer studies have examined receptionists' relationship with other members of the practice team. Those studies that have examined this dynamic have tended to examine the ways that receptionists were valued by GPs, with Copeman and Van Zwanenberg (1988), for example, asking whether receptionists were 'poorly valued and underpaid?' An exception to this is a recent ethnographic study examining the repeat prescribing routines of four general practices in England by Swinglehurst *et al.* (2011) which showed that receptionists played a significant role in ensuring the quality and safety of repeat prescribing by making extensive use of tacit knowledge and situated judgements to bridge the gap between the formal organisational routine and the actual routine as it was played out in practice. However, given the central roles of both receptionists and GPs in this work and the potentially differing worldviews, logics, priorities and understandings of what constitutes safe, reliable care between these team members, it is equally important to develop a more detailed understanding of the nature of the coordination work that is undertaken between these professions and their relative contributions to repeat prescribing safety. Furthermore, given the cultural variation that exists across UK general practices as independent businesses (Grant *et al.* 2014), it will also be important to examine contextual differences between practices in greater detail across both formal and informal routines. This chapter ethnographically examines the formal and informal work employed by GPs and receptionists to safely conduct repeat prescribing work in UK general practice using Strauss's (1985) concept of 'articulation work' across a range of general practice contexts.

Methods

The study was conducted during a Medical Research Council Population Health Scientist Fellowship held by SG (2009–13). The overall aim of the study was to examine the ways in which quality and safety were achieved across a range of organisational routines in UK general practice using ethnographic methods. This chapter focuses on the collaborative work required by general practice teams to achieve safety in their repeat prescribing routines.

Sampling and data collection
The study was conducted in NHS Scotland and NHS England from January 2011–April 2014 using a multi-site case study design across 8 urban and rural general practices (pseudonymised as 'Practice 1', 'Practice 2', 'Practice 3', etc.). Practices were purposively selected on the basis of their size (smaller with ~4,000 patients or larger with ~9.000 patients), socioeconomic deprivation of the population served (affluent, mixed or deprived), and location (urban and small town/rural) (Table 1). Data collection was in two phases, with an in-depth ethnographic study conducted in Practices 1–4 over a 24-month period in 2011/12, followed by more rapid ethnographic methods involving one week of fieldwork per practice applied in Practices 5–8 in 2013/14 focusing on specific organisational routines, including repeat prescribing.

A multi-sited ethnographic approach was adopted combining observation of everyday practice with interviews and documentary analysis. SG undertook 1,787 hours of ethnographic fieldwork from January 2011–April 2014. Informed consen.. was obtained from each practice team member prior to fieldwork commencing, and it was repeatedly explained that the researcher was interested in learning about the organisational culture, systems and processes of the practice and not in assessing individuals' performance. Fieldwork was undertaken with clinical, managerial and administrative staff during normal working hours in reception areas, back offices, consulting rooms, administrative offices, meeting rooms, coffee rooms and corridors. Detailed handwritten fieldnotes were made in full view of informants, and later transcribed for coding. Narratives were elicited from staff as they worked by the researcher asking them to talk through what they were doing and to 'think aloud' as they conducted their everyday work. These narratives were recorded with permission and later transcribed and coded. Documentary analysis of relevant written protocols (where available) and patient information leaflets from each practice was also conducted.

Towards the end of fieldwork in each practice, 62 semi-structured interviews were conducted by SG with GPs, practice nurses, practice managers and administrative staff (Table 2). Interviewees were selected based on observation of their work, and gave informed consent

Table 1   *Practice characteristics and duration of fieldwork*

Practice no.	Country	Practice size	Practice urban/rural location	Practice socioeconomic deprivation	Duration of fieldwork
1	Scotland	~4000	Urban	Mixed	In-depth
2	Scotland	~9000	Urban	Deprived	In-depth
3	Scotland	~5000	Urban	Mixed	In-depth
4	Scotland	~8000	Rural	Affluent	In-depth
5	England	~5000	Urban	Mixed	Rapid
6	England	~6000	Rural	Affluent	Rapid
7	Scotland	~9000	Urban	Deprived	Rapid
8	Scotland	~8000	Rural	Affluent	Rapid

to participate before the interview commenced. The interview topics included: the interviewee's role within the practice; the practice organisational structure and culture; interviewee's descriptions of each organisational routine that they were involved in; the key ways in which they collaborated with other practice team members; and key strengths and weaknesses of each organisational routine in terms of patient safety. The interviews lasted 60 minutes on average, and were recorded and transcribed verbatim.

Table 2   *Practice interviewees by profession*

Practice no.	GP	Practice nurse	Practice manager	Administrative staff	Total
1	2	2	1	3	8
2	2	2	1	3	8
3	2	2	1	2	7
4	2	2	1	3	8
5	2	1	1	3	7
6	2	1	1	3	7
7	2	2	1	2	7
8	3	2	1	4	10
Total	17	14	8	23	62

Analytical approach

Analysis drew on the concept of articulation work, which Strauss (1985) developed to examine the nature of collaboration between professionals and the knowledge and resources that are necessary to conduct such work. Articulation work refers to 'the specifics of putting together tasks, task sequences, task clusters – even aligning larger units of work such as lines of work or subprojects – in the service of work flow' (Strauss 1988: 164). Since actors have to continuously adjust and realign their own individual actions in coordination with those of other actors, collaborative work requires the continuous readjustment of planned courses of action rather than a singular, linear course of action directed by formal rules and norms (Fjuk *et al.* 1997). Articulation work is the adjustment and alignment that is necessary to make organisational work happen, and individual activities cannot therefore be understood without taking into account the socio-cultural settings within which they take place.

Strauss (1993: 54) emphasises the temporal dimension of articulation work through the concept of 'trajectories', which are 'the course of any experienced phenomenon as it evolves over time' in ways that are not always predictable. Actors within a given trajectory have to establish and negotiate 'what work is to be done, to what standards, in what space, during what time period, with what resources, by whom, and with what payback' (Strauss 1993: 89). Strauss (1985) refers to the totality of tasks conducted over a period of time as an 'arc of work' which has a specific temporal trajectory, within which individuals have to constantly renegotiate their practices in the face of unexpected interactions and events. The trajectories of particular arcs of work are both multiple and intersecting and may be conducted sequentially, concurrently, or in phases, with specific practices being prioritised and structuring the execution of other coordinative activities (Fjuk *et al.* 1997, Strauss 1985). Strauss's concept of 'arc of work' resonated strongly with that of the repeat prescribing routine, which comprises a range of interconnected tasks conducted by different professionals over a specific period of time.

A further key feature of articulation work is the distinction that Strauss (1985) makes between formal and informal work where, in order to reduce the complexity of effort involved in articulation work, teams employ a range of mechanisms to standardise and simplify this work to render it predictable (e.g. standard operating procedures (SOPs) and protocols). Alongside this formal 'upper level' articulation work, organisational routines also contain informal elements that 'modif[y] action to accommodate unexpected contingencies' (Star 1991: 275) which are less well documented and/or officially authorised. Mesman (2010: 111) describes this as 'diagnostic work', which involves 'the recognition of the overall task structure, the ability 'to read' the conduct of co-participants and the identification of opportunities for interaction' in order for actors to 'act in the same present'. Individuals therefore need to be tuned into each other's tasks in order to recognise which actions should be adjusted, in what way, and when.

Finally, articulation work also has strong spatial dimension, which has been developed by Bardram and Bossen (2005) through the concept of 'mobility work'. Bardram and Bossen (2005: 136, italics in original) write: 'Mobility work designates the work needed to achieve the *right configuration of people, resources, knowledge and place* in order to carry out tasks at a certain point in time'. As a spatial complement to the temporally-focused SOPs, Bardram and Bossen (2005) developed the concept of 'standard operating configurations' (SOCs), which are 'a spatial setup fostering easy cooperation because of common knowledge and agreement as to use and navigation' (Bardram and Bossen 2005:138). Just like SOPs, SOCs provide a standard spatial arrangement of work practices.

Over the years, many studies of health and community work have proved the analytical strength of the concept of 'articulation work', particularly when applied in conjunction with a practice-based approach (Nicolini 2012) in which social phenomena are understood as being continually (re)created through active human agency (e.g. Allen 2014, Hampson and Junor 2005). For example, in her study of the invisible work of nurses, Allen (2014) employed a practice-based approach (Nicolini 2012) to distinguish between several forms of articulation work, including temporal, material, and integrative articulation. Others, like Fjuk *et al.* (1997), combined the work of Strauss with activity theory to examine the external factors and artefacts that influence actions. Our analysis underlines the added value of these and other theoretical elaborations to the concept of 'articulation work'.

Both fieldnotes and interviews were annotated with observational and theoretical notes and shared between the research team. This provided an opportunity for multidisciplinary reflection and enriched enquiry. The researcher (SG) read the interview transcripts to become familiar with the data. Preliminary themes were identified through scrutiny of initial transcripts and a coding framework was subsequently developed that was embedded in the data collected (Mays and Pope 1995), with Strauss's concept of articulation work used as a sensitising concept during the course of the analysis. This framework was consistently applied to the remaining transcripts using NVivo 8 (QSR International, Doncaster, Australia) software. The framework was refined according to emerging themes across the eight practices as the fieldwork developed. The modified framework was then reapplied to all transcripts, and this constant comparative method continued until no further categories emerged.

Results

Doctors and non-medical prescribers commonly issue prescriptions during face-to-face encounters, but most prescribing takes place without the patient being present, and starts with a request for a prescription made by phone, in writing, or at the reception desk. These requests can be for drugs that have been authorised for repeat issuing without a consultation ('repeats'), or for drugs which the patent has never had before, or drugs which the patient has had before but which have not been formally authorised for repeat issuing ('acutes'). As the demand for repeat prescriptions has increased over the past decades (Petty *et al.* 2014), practices have had to evolve these systems to manage this growing volume of work by balancing the rapid turnaround of prescription requests with the quality and safety of prescribing.

Managing the growing volume of repeat prescribing

Clinical professional control of prescribing relies on claims that this is the only way to ensure appropriate and safe use of potentially dangerous medicines, and is made concrete by the requirement for an individual qualified clinician (usually a GP) to sign each prescription and take responsibility for its issue. Key tasks in the repeat prescribing arc of work therefore included the management of requests and the printing of the correct prescriptions by receptionists, the delivery of a bundle of routine repeat prescriptions to GPs for signing with separate bundles of other requests to GPs to decide whether to issue, and the delivery of signed prescriptions or requests for further information or consultation back to patients. The volume of work involved was challenging for all eight practices to deliver:

> It can be a huge bundle of stuff. You know, you could quite easily spend two or more hours doing repeat prescribing every day. Some days it's huge … It usually breaks your spirits quite significantly. (Practice 4, GP2)

In the past, GPs often only signed repeat prescriptions for 'their' patients, but in all eight practices, all routine repeat prescriptions were signed by the daily 'duty doctor' in order to assure turnaround within 48 hours. However, the volume of prescriptions requiring signing made it impossible for the duty GP to double-check the details of every repeat prescription in the clinical record before signing them:

> The vast majority are ones that are just routine and will be just signed. I mean when I say routine, obviously they have to be re-authorised every so often, but if they're authorised and it's all okay then it's usually just a question of signing it. (Practice 3, GP2)

Within the context of increased pressure on GPs' time, key requirements of the repeat prescribing system – careful checking of the accuracy and appropriateness of the request vs. rapid turnaround – compete for attention in a resource-constrained environment. GPs therefore relied on receptionists to appropriately issue and print prescriptions for signing with little further review, and to flag non-routine prescriptions for GPs' special attention. This socio-material configuration acted as a replacement for safety work that was fundamentally a GP clinical task, and required GPs to have to trust in the integrity of the repeat prescribing system and in the expertise of the receptionist:

> You've just got to assume that the system is working. But it's a big task and it's ever-growing and there's no way of checking each and every script, you just can't do it. It's huge, I mean it's massive now. When I started 27 years ago it was a small task and there was a small bundle everyday but now it's probably 5 times as much as it was. (Practice 4, GP1)

Three of the eight practices had no written protocol that specified how the 'system' was meant to work (Practices 1, 3 and 7) and in these practices, repeat prescribing was regarded as specialised work to be done by one full-time and long-serving expert receptionist in collaboration with the GPs, making a written protocol redundant (Table 3). The perceived safety

Table 3 *Practice organisation of repeat prescribing*

	Practice 1 (NHS Scotland)	Practice 2 (NHS Scotland)	Practice 3 (NHS Scotland)	Practice 4 (NHS Scotland)	Practice 5 (NHS England)	Practice 6 (NHS England)	Practice 7 (NHS Scotland)	Practice 8 (NHS Scotland)
Written protocol?	No	Yes. Written by head receptionist	No	Yes. Written by head receptionist	Yes. Six pages written by GP and intended to be used by the whole team	Yes. Two pages written by practice manager and intended to delineate receptionist tasks	No	Yes. Written by head receptionist
Administrative responsibility for repeat prescribing	Single receptionist	Multi-tasking team	Single receptionist	Single receptionist	Multi-tasking team	Multi-tasking team	Single receptionist	Multi-tasking team
Practice ethos	Traditional family practice	Modern business	Traditional family practice	Modern business	Traditional family practice	Traditional family practice	Modern business	Modern business
Practice building	NHS-owned health centre with space rented by the practice	Purpose-built modern health centre owned by the practice	NHS-owned health centre with space rented by the practice	Purpose-built modern health centre owned by the practice	Converted Victorian house owned by the practice	Purpose-built modern health centre owned by the practice	NHS-owned health centre with space rented by the practice	NHS-owned health centre with space rented by the practice

of this way of working lay in these experienced receptionists' accumulated knowledge of the clinical IT system, of drug names and doses, and of the 'regular' patients who were taking many medicines.

The remaining five practices had formal repeat prescribing protocols, written by one of the GPs (Practice 5), the practice manager (Practice 6), or the head receptionist (Practices 2, 4 and 8). These were primarily intended to be used by reception teams, who shared the repeat prescribing work to varying degrees. In Practice 4, repeat prescribing was also the responsibility of one receptionist, but in the other four practices with written protocols, it was a team-based task that practice managers had increasingly formalised as the volume of repeat prescribing had increased. In these four practices, repeat prescribing work was something that all members of the reception team were expected to have expertise in. Although it was acknowledged that there were safety risks involved in using less expert individuals and in the subsequent need for repeated handovers of complex information, this was considered less risky than relying on a single individual, which posed problems if that person was absent or left the practice.

Despite the close association between practices organising repeat prescribing work around teams and having written protocols, the protocols were not observed to be used during repeat prescribing work by anyone in the five practices, with many staff claiming never to have seen them or saying that they were part of their introductory pack but that they had never been read. Rather, GP and receptionist accounts of repeat prescribing work emphasised tacit knowledge as forming the basis of how repeat prescribing work was conducted on an every-day basis. Involved staff would readily provide detailed accounts of the whole arc of work, which included descriptions of the tasks that were required to be completed, the order that they should be done in, and the professionals who were involved in completing each task. In the practices that had them, protocols were largely used for the initial training of new staff, but had limited use beyond this.

While the same key elements of the arc of work were described by participants in all eight practices, practices varied in the order in which these elements were said to happen, and the combinations of staff involved at each stage. Initial interview descriptions also largely described what was intended to happen with routine prescription requests rather than how the whole range of requests were managed. Non-participant observation and think aloud interviews revealed a body of non-routine, 'invisible' articulation work (Allen 2014, Hampson and Junor 2005, Star 1991) conducted by GPs and receptionists to ensure delivery of the repeat prescribing arc of work. Space precludes a detailed description of all the work done, and so we focus on how requests were initially managed by receptionists in terms of those routinely issued versus those flagged for GPs' attention, how routine work was transferred from one member of the team to another, and how non-routine or urgent work was managed using a range of interruption practices.

Initial management of requests by receptionists

A core receptionist task in all of the practices was to distinguish between prescription requests that were authorised and legitimate 'repeats' that simply required GPs signing and prescriptions that required further attention from the duty GP, either because there were fac-tors that made an authorised repeat problematic (for example, an early request), or because the request was for an acute prescription which was not authorised for regular issue. How-ever, an important difference between the practices studied was in terms of the range of items that the GPs permitted the receptionists to issue and print.

In some practices, receptionists were only allowed to print items that were formally set up in the IT system as authorised 'repeats'. In Practices 4 and 6, receptionists were only allowed to issue and print items that were listed in the repeats section and so pre-authorised for regular issue, although the reasons given for this differed. Practice 6 was a rural dispensing practice (i.e. also took the pharmacists' role in dispensing drugs), and the GPs limited receptionist discretion since they perceived that not having an independent pharmacist involved in dispensing meant that any errors introduced earlier in the process were less likely to be detected. In Practice 4, the same tight control on what receptionists could issue was justified in the context of the GPs' pride in being a traditional family practice where GPs looked after 'their' patients. The GPs therefore dealt with all repeat prescription requests themselves during their shared morning coffee break, dividing the work between themselves based on who knew the patient best to both minimise error and provide personal care.

In the remaining practices, the receptionists were allowed to issue and print a limited range of 'acute' items beyond those formally authorised for repeat prescription. For example, the experienced specialist computer operator in Practice 1 had a list of acute drugs that she could issue attached to the wall, although these still required case-by-case checking by a GP, achieved by her attaching a yellow sticky note to the front of the printed prescription asking the duty GP if they were 'OK to give?'. While GPs acknowledged that this introduced some risk into the system since GPs could sign such a prescription without opening the record, the intent of this was to reduce the demands on GP time while ensuring that potentially problematic prescriptions were made obvious to the GP. In other practices, receptionists had fewer formal limits on what they could issue. In Practice 7, for example, the highly experienced 'repeats guru' was allowed to issue and print the widest range of medications of any practice, which was justified in terms of the experience that she had of both patients and the names and doses of different kinds of medication. She would thus frequently issue and print acute requests for GPs to sign and return to her without much oversight, which the practice felt was required to manage the very high volume of prescription requests made by the socioeconomically deprived population the practice served.

Across all of the practices, receptionists had to make decisions about how to direct GPs' attention to the problematic requests. Methods varied between practices and between individual receptionists in the same practice in terms of how this was done, with sticky notes, highlighter pens, ballpoint pens, notebooks and paperclips used to efficiently draw GPs' attention to elements of the request that the receptionist judged problematic. Receptionists devoted considerable time in all eight practices to this work, thus simplifying complex information to minimise the time GPs spent dealing with each problematic request.

In summary, timely management of the high volume of repeat prescribing requests in all practices required the delegation by GPs of key safety tasks to receptionists in order to save GP time, including safe identification of which drugs the patient was requesting, initial judgement about whether the request was an unproblematic repeat, and clear signalling to the GP of problematic requests. Practices varied in terms of what receptionists were permitted to do and how they simplified the following stage of work for GPs, but despite these differences, the repeat prescribing arc of work in all of these practices included large sets of tasks for the receptionists to undertake. Across each of the practices, receptionists played a key role in the simplification of the work of GPs and there was mutual coordination of each other's tasks across the repeat prescribing arc of work. The following section examines the transfer of prescriptions between GPs and receptionists in greater detail.

Transferring practices for routine repeat prescribing work
The efficient and effective transfer of tasks, documents and information between different members of the team was central to repeat prescribing work, but largely undocumented in the protocols that existed. A key role of the receptionists was to ensure that the 'pile' of

standard repeat prescriptions was in the correct place at the correct time for the duty GP to collect and sign. Timing and positioning of the pile were crucial in order to constitute and maintain an arc of work to create a set of signed prescriptions for giving to the patient or pharmacist. The alignment of the different elements required both formal and informal articulation work with both temporal and spatial dimensions. Temporal articulation (Bardram 2000) refers to the articulation work that aims to position actions in the right moment and order. What is considered to be the right moment is based upon the prioritizing of different interdependent lines of work (e.g. seeing patients, doing house visits, the 48-hour turnaround of prescriptions). An important element in the temporal articulation work is the organising effect of deadlines. Here deadlines act as temporal markers within the overall flow of time. Rather than acting as a constraint, they act as a positive temporal beacon that one can focus on and align other activities around.

The transfer of prescriptions from the receptionist to the GP also required 'mobility work' (Bardram and Bossen 2005), with each practice having its own system for ensuring that this process took place smoothly and on time. For example, throughout the morning in Practice 2, the receptionist would accumulate a pile of standard repeats in a wire tray on her desk, and ensure that by 2 pm the pile was transferred to a purple folder in the duty doctor document tray for collection. In contrast, in Practice 1, the receptionist would continually bring prescriptions from her office to the table in the GPs' coffee room next door for the duty doctor to sign whenever they could throughout the day. The different approaches adopted by these practices constitute distinct modes of ordering (Law 1994). The receptionist in Practice 2 constituted part of a chain of intermediaries, with the trays and folders acting as a passageway that provided a trajectory for the prescription to travel from her desk to the GP. In other words, piles, trays and folders were 'coordinating artefacts' (Allen 2014: 61) that supported the arc of work. This consecutive mode of ordering differs from the one in Practice 1 where the mode of ordering was not compartmentalized but a continuous flow of work.

GPs were responsible for the timely return of signed repeats back to the receptionists, but how this was achieved varied between practices and between GPs within the same practice. In Practice 1, the duty GP would carry signed prescriptions back to the receptionist's office next door, whereas the duty GP in Practice 3 would hand them to the receptionist at the front desk who would then sort them into an alphabetically-arranged box for patients to collect. While the receptionists usually had strict deadlines to adhere to for their own cluster of tasks pre and post-GP signing, the GPs had greater autonomy and less pressure to be punctual, which then often required additional complex mobility work on the part of the receptionists to retrieve the prescriptions from the GPs. For example, in Practice 4 the duty GP was responsible for signing repeat prescriptions but if other work prevented them from doing this, prescriptions were shared equally between all of the GPs during coffee break to enable the receptionists 'to get the prescriptions moving' (Practice 4, Receptionist 2). However, this then created a retrieval problem for receptionists because it was unclear which GP had which scripts:

> Some days you find they have shared them out and other days you've got them all back from the one person, you know? It isn't great for us as we've lost track of where everything has gone and we just have to keep going back to them and saying 'look these scripts haven't come back, we had them on Tuesday, this is by Thursday' you know … You have to be assertive. (Practice 4, Receptionist 1)

In Practice 8, the receptionist would 'bundle [the scripts] out evenly' (Receptionist 1) across all of the GPs' trays at the back of reception so that they all 'got their quota'. While some GPs returned their morning prescriptions at lunchtime and then collected their next pile for signing, others returned prescriptions gradually between patients during their afternoon surgery creating delays for receptionists in making them available for collection.

In summary, this section has shown that even the most routine repeat prescribing work requires articulation work to ensure that it runs as smoothly and simply as possible. While the transfer of repeat prescription requests is a spatial task (the transfer of documents from A to B) requiring mobility work by both receptionists and GPs, it is also highly dependent on temporal aspects of articulation work in order for this spatial articulation be achieved at the right moment. This temporal element has different implications for receptionists and GPs: while receptionists had fixed deadlines that acted as planning devices, GPs had greater temporal freedom, which partly related to their position of authority within the general practice organisation. The following section examines the least routine element of repeat prescribing, which is the role of interruptions in the achievement of this arc of work.

Interrupting practices for non-routine repeat prescribing work
The repeat prescribing arc of work is only one of many arcs of work happening simultaneously in all practices, including the opening, scanning and management of letters and test results, making appointments, and managing the constant flow of patients coming to the reception desk for multiple reasons. GPs and receptionists in all eight practices therefore regularly interrupted each other's work in order to complete their own work. The patient safety literature has tended to focus on the risks posed by interruptions, with distractions, for example, said to lead to transcription and other errors, or the non-completion of tasks. However, in all eight practices, interruptions were essential opportunities to efficiently interact with colleagues. The following fieldnote extract illustrates the kinds of interruptions that can take place for receptionists on a day-to-day basis:

09:31: Receptionist 1 brought another large handful of repeat prescription requests through to her office from the blue plastic box on the front desk of main reception area. This bundle was as large as the one that she had brought through earlier this morning when had she collected her first batch of requests from the box at 08:10. 'That's Monday mornings for you!' she exclaimed as she placed them down on her desk in front of her computer … The rest of the repeat prescriptions pile from earlier that morning were still there, but she had decided to collect this more recent bundle whilst she was in the main reception asking the Duty Doctor to sign an urgent prescription request for a patient who had just been discharged from hospital.

09:34: Receptionist 1 took the first repeats request off the top of the pile and read through the key elements of the request … She checked that the items were on repeats on the patient's record, that they were not over-ordering or due a medication review, and then authorised the request by printing off the prescription.

09:38: Just as she began working on [the next prescription request], Receptionist 4 came into the office and said 'Sorry to bother you, but Mr [name of patient]'s wife has just come in and handed in an urgent request for his pain killers – do you think you could just print it off now to save him waiting till tomorrow?' Receptionist 1 said she would as he was a 'poor soul' and placed the script that she had been working on to the left hand side of her keyboard with her pen on top to mark the place before printing off the prescription. Receptionist 4 thanked her and stuck her head out of the door to look down the corridor, saying that she would 'catch' GP2 and ask him to sign it right away as he was 'just going into the main reception to get his mail'. (Practice 1, fieldnotes, 14.09.12)

Across all eight practices, the 'catching' of colleagues was necessary to ensure that all required work including repeat prescribing was done safely and effectively. On the basis of her ethnographic findings, Carroll (2009: 160) stresses that 'being available, being interrupted, interacting with colleagues and taking advantage of opportunistic communications, are fundamental to the progression of patient treatment and to redevelop effective daily work plans'. Although interruptions seem to be an indication of non-order or even chaos, Carroll writes that interruptions should not carry a solely negative connotation as they should be understood as a regular and characteristic feature of the work that also positively contribute to the flux of everyday work. Within the context of repeat prescribing, these non-ordered interactions allowed for adaptive decision-making regarding patients and work planning. There were many ways in which 'catching' could be done, including through electronic messaging, waiting for opportunities as clinical staff moved around the building, hovering in corridors or outside consulting rooms until someone was free, phoning them, or going to their workspace or consulting room. In other words, the permeability of time and space afforded order to the repeat prescribing routine and also enabled this order to be constantly updated (Carroll 2009: 161).

In some of the practices, the GPs actively encouraged the receptionist doing repeat prescribing to 'catch' them to discuss queries face-to-face because they perceived this to be more efficient. For example, in Practice 8, the GPs had deliberately placed the house visits book behind the repeats desk so that the receptionists had a continual flow of GPs available to 'catch' to complete non-standard work including repeat prescribing. The GPs also used this shared space to 'catch' receptionists to complete their own non-standard tasks such as phoning the hospital to resolve a query. Similarly, the shared coffee room in Practice 5 was situated behind the front office next to the repeat prescribing desk. This was intended to encourage the doctors to spend time in this area and facilitate informal and problem-solving interactions with nursing and reception staff, as the following fieldnote illustrates:

> One of the young female salaried GPs comes into the reception area to collect her lunch from the fridge and make a cup of tea. She had been talking to one of the practice nurses sitting at the seating area about her forthcoming wedding plans. Receptionist 3 is at the repeats desk and asks her if she can ask her a 'quick question'. The GP comes across and the receptionist tells her that a female patient of 67 yrs had just phoned in requesting morphine. The receptionist tells the GP that the patient 'sounded like she was in a lot of pain' and decided not to write it down in the black 'problem scripts' book, as the request wouldn't be dealt with until lunchtime. The receptionist asks what she should do. The GP tells her 'We don't normally do this, but this patient is elderly and in lots of pain, so I think it's OK to fax the morphine prescription to the pharmacist'. (Fieldnotes, Practice 5, 09.07.13)

For more urgent requests, receptionists would more actively seek to locate any or a particular GP. This was variously referred to as 'hovering' or 'lurking' around the practice corridors until they 'caught' a suitable doctor that could respond to their request. Iedema et al (2006) explain how this 'corridor work' turns a marginal space such as the corridor into a site of intense productivity that is an important resource for healthcare teams:

> This is a unique site where final decisions can be held in abeyance and where uncertainties and provisional decisions can co-exist; a space where the fixities of hierarchy and specialization can be attenuated if not suspended, and a space where people can agree to work around rules and regulations; in short, a space where tasks and

positionings become sufficiently provisional, flexible and negotiable to enable clinicians to weave the complexity of emerging facets of clinical practice into a workable and productive unfolding. (Iedema *et al.* 2006: 238)

Partly to reduce the risks associated with interruptions, the repeats receptionists in Practices 1 and 7 worked in specially-designated individual offices. This required them to employ different tactics to catch clinical staff for non-standard repeat prescribing work. In Practice 1, for example, the repeats receptionist would keep all problem scripts in a small pile to the side of her desk and 'catch' GPs or nurses opportunistically as they entered the office. However, if she required urgent advice or a signature, she would often 'keep an eye on the window' of the office that faced the main corridor to the GPs' consulting rooms and 'catch' a GP as they walked past. Across all of the practices, receptionists would regularly check the practice appointment system on their computer screen to see which GP was free at that moment, with many deliberately targeting specific GPs that they knew were more amenable to interruptions of particular types of request:

The girls at reception, we know which doctors would sign an urgent script, you know, without grumbling. So we kind of watch the screen to see who's going to be the next one up and then go down the corridor to catch them. If we have an urgent prescription that comes through, then we go tap on the door of a doctor and just say 'Please'. (Practice 8, Receptionist 1)

Some practices had created defined time for lower urgency catching, for example through having a number of 2-minute long appointment slots in the morning and afternoon for GPs to examine any 'problem queries'. This reduced interruption of GPs, but also meant that receptionists knew when particular tasks were due to be completed.

In other practices, the building layout mitigated against informal interaction, with Practices 2 and 4 for example having a separate GP corridor that was located at the opposite end of the practice from the reception. In these practices where there were fewer opportunities for face-to-face catching, there was a greater reliance by receptionists on electronic messaging and telephone calls, notably in Practices 2, 4, 6 and 7. Electronic messaging in particular had been actively developed in all four of these practices in order to create a clear audit trail for tasks being transferred (e.g. receptionists had to initial each communication for audit purposes) and to minimise time spent physically locating one another. The GPs in Practice 4, for example, described themselves as being at the cutting edge of technology, and receptionists made extensive use of instant messaging 'bubbles' which appeared instantly in the middle of the recipient's screen and facilitated rapid responses to simple queries. For example:

Receptionist 3 sends a 'bubble' [a message on the practice IT system that instantly appears in the middle of the recipient's screen] to GP2 saying '[first name of GP], pt forgot to ask for an rx for Priadel 200 mg. Could you write an rx and send to chemist? Thanks [initial of receptionist]'. GP2 responds several minutes later with: 'Do not issue. Make an appointment with patient to see me [initials of GP]'. The receptionist then phoned the patient to ask him to make an appointment with the doctor to discuss their request further. (Practice 4, fieldnotes, 15.02.12; pt = patient, rx = prescription)

In summary, while interruptions have frequently been presented in the patient safety literature as risky activities that are conducive to errors, this section has shown that interrupting the routine flow of tasks in an arc of work was frequently employed by GPs and receptionists as a way to prioritise and manage urgent, higher-risk work.

Discussion

The application of Strauss's (1985) concept of articulation work to examine the formal and informal work required to safely conduct repeat prescribing work in UK general practice has revealed the central role of informal spatio-temporal re-adjustment and re-alignment by GPs and receptionists as positive, proactive safety solutions to continually relocate vulnerability in time and space. Through the lens of articulation work and the application of ethnographic methods, this study has also revealed the central role of the informal, invisible practices of general practice receptionists, with informal, cross-hierarchical communication often more effective than formal structures of communication. This discussion examines these issues in greater detail.

The application of articulation work to examine medication safety in UK general practice has enabled the exploration of the relationship between the formal, visible elements of repeat prescribing work alongside more informal, invisible elements, and their respective roles in the achievement of repeat prescribing safety. While some of the general practices in this study had written protocols that outlined a simplified version of the technical aspects of the process, the complexity of the work involved in coordinating repeat prescribing alongside the other arcs of work that were taking place concurrently (e.g. test ordering, patient consultations, opening mail) rendered such formal documents inadequate as practical navigational guides for GPs or receptionists. As recent studies have shown (Grol *et al.* 2008, Iedema 2009, Mesman 2009, 2010, 2011, Rowley and Waring 2011, Macrae 2014), the application of rules, guidelines, regulations and protocols for patient safety improvement will never fully eradicate the imperfect and contingent nature of everyday work practices and the presence of risk and vulnerability therein. The analytical lens of articulation work and the adoption of a practice-based approach (Nicolini 2012) has illuminated not just the risks, vulnerabilities and potential errors inherent in repeat prescribing work (e.g. transcription errors, communication errors), but also the local, informal resources of resilience and strength that were employed by practice team members in the achievement of repeat prescribing safety. Space was therefore both a challenge (invisibility when receptionists were located in separate rooms) as well as a solution (corridor work). Time was also both a challenge (shortage of time for GPs to conduct every element of the high-volume, safety-critical administrative work) as well as a solution (interruptions). By making explicit the mundane, local routines across the eight practices, we were able to 'exnovate' (Mesman 2011) (i.e. make visible) the already existing local competencies that were routinely employed but invisible to both rationalised models of organisational analysis (Star and Strauss 1999) and team members themselves because they were used every day. An analytical focus on visible and invisible work proved to be a powerful tool for developing a more nuanced understanding of both the vulnerabilities and strengths of repeat prescribing configurations across a range of organisational contexts (Hampson and Junor 2005).

This study was conducted across eight general practices in Scotland and England, which enabled a comparative examination of the strengths and vulnerabilities of different repeat prescribing routines. While the formal stages of the repeat prescribing routine were broadly similar across the eight practices, each had adopted different context-specific solutions that spanned organisational (e.g. multi-tasking team vs. individual repeats 'gurus'), temporal (e.g. fixed deadlines vs. flexible timings), and spatial (e.g. placing prescriptions to be signed in a tray for GPs to collect vs. placing them directly in the coffee room) spheres of practice. This study showed that across the eight practices, the different spatio-temporal configurations that were employed illuminated different organisational and individual strengths, while at the same time displacing different vulnerabilities across space and time. Thus, while the presence of multi-tasking teams, for example, reduced the risks associated with concentrating receptionist expertise in the hands of one person (e.g. during holidays or if that person left), it also increased the risk of error associated with multiple handovers. While the uniqueness of individual practice systems may in part reflect the status of general practices as small, independent businesses owned by GP partnerships with unique socio-cultural traits (Grant *et al.* 2014), by examining the informal articulation work involved in repeat prescribing work, we were also able to develop a more nuanced understanding of the complex trade-offs that different practice teams made through the range of approaches that were adopted based on organisational strengths and weaknesses and the application of tacit knowledge by key individuals across this arc of work (The Health Foundation 2014).

Alongside the complexities of coordinating the individual tasks within an arc of work, Strauss (1985: 9) highlights the nature of the interrelationship between the multiple arcs of work that take place simultaneously within an organisational setting, with 'one receiving more organisational priority than another at a given phase'. Within the patient safety literature, such intersections are frequently reported as challenges to patient safety and a key cause of error (e.g. Avery *et al.* 2013). However, in this study we found that these intersections were purposively employed by GPs and receptionists as opportunities for the achievement and maintenance of repeat prescribing safety in the face of an increasingly challenging workload. The completion of urgent work frequently resulted in the creation of impromptu spatial configurations across the practices beyond the SOCs that were typically employed by practices. Thus, interruptions provided informal, impromptu opportunities for GPs and receptionists to communicate and prioritise tasks in multi-purpose, 'liminal' (Iedema *et al.* 2006) spaces such as corridors, coffee rooms and back offices, and so prevent the arc of work from stalling. Similarly, deadlines were not simply engaged with as closures to particular tasks but rather as supportive structures for receptionists to coordinate the repeat prescribing arc of work whilst taking into account other arcs of work that interfered with its completion (see also Allen 2014). IT was also frequently employed by practices to crosscut spatial boundaries, particularly in practices where impromptu meeting opportunities were limited. These 'latent resources of safety' have been described by Mesman (2011) as taken-for-granted 'hidden competencies' that are held by individuals and teams. Time and space were therefore creatively, flexibly and positively employed by practices as tools of resilience rather than being fixed obstacles to be overcome.

Recent writers have emphasised that a key strength of articulation work has been in highlighting the informal, less visible elements of professional work (e.g. Hampson and Junor 2005, Postma *et al.* 2014, Star 1991). As was the case in Allen's (2014) study of UK secondary care, no practice team member was formally responsible for overseeing the repeat prescribing arc of work in any of the practices in this study. On a formal level, the GPs were responsible for authorising each prescription through signing them, and there were a range of intersecting hierarchical elements to the relationship between GPs and receptionists: receptionists were employees of the GP partnership, and it was the GPs who considered themselves to have 'overall authority' for the patients. Like nursing (Allen 2014), receptionist work is also highly gendered, with most receptionists being female and working class. While these underlying hierarchical features were present across all of the practices, this ethnographic study has also revealed the dynamic nature of the role boundary between GPs and receptionists, which varied depending on the nature of articulation work being conducted.

While GPs' formal authority for repeat prescribing was physically enacted through their signing of each repeat prescription, it was the receptionists who were responsible for the initiation and overall coordination of the repeat prescribing arc of work. Gherardi (2006) writes that arcs of work are multiple and intersecting and with differing degrees of complexity or 'density'. Coordinating the overall navigation of multiple intersecting tasks with varying degrees of complexity required a great deal of creativity, flexibility and initiative on the part of receptionists in order to achieve the correct configuration of team members and artefacts in the right place at the right time (Allen 2014, Hampson and Junor 2005, Suchman 1987). The high volume of repeat prescription requests and the urgent nature of many of these requests meant that GPs placed a great deal of trust and authority in receptionists to ensure that prescriptions were filtered correctly. For example, receptionists had the authority to re-authorise repeat medication and authorise certain 'acute' requests in practices where the repeats volume was particularly high. Allen (2014: 4) writes that invisible work lies 'at the heart of politics about what will count as work'. An examination of repeat prescribing invisible work has shown that receptionists were a key locus of strength in the repeat prescribing routine across all of the practices. However, due to the mundane, 'routine' and most importantly invisible nature of this work, it is rarely acknowledged and infrequently examined in depth. Building on Suchman's (2000) challenge to the dichotomy between 'knowledge' and 'routine' work, this study has therefore also highlighted the importance of tacit knowledge, practical reasoning and situational judgements on the part of administrative staff which are crucial for the maintenance of quality and safety in healthcare organisations.

Conclusion

This chapter has examined the different ways in which safety is achieved within a high-volume routine in UK general practice. As risky sociotechnical environments (Owen *et al.* 2009), healthcare organisations such as hospitals and general practices are inherently fallible, with technical and communication breakdowns, failures and incidents intrinsic characteristics of everyday work. The application of Strauss's (1985) concept of articulation work provided an effective analytical lens through which to examine the formal and informal ways in which repeat prescribing safety was achieved across eight UK general practice contexts and the strengths and vulnerabilities that exist across different practice socio-cultural contexts.

A recent report by The Health Foundation (2014) has highlighted the fundamental importance of understanding and taking into account internal organisational context in examining and implementing quality improvement work. In this report, (ibid.: 96) defines 'practical wisdom' (i.e. experience-based knowledge) and 'conjectural knowledge' (i.e. contextually-based stealth in achieving one's purpose) as essential elements of successful quality improvement work and evaluations. In this study, the application of ethnographic methods enabled an in-depth examination of each general practice context as well as the 'practical wisdom' and 'conjectural knowledge' employed by both GPs and receptionists in the achievement of prescribing safety. Of particular value has been the practice-based insight (Nicolini 2012) that articulation work provided into the informal, invisible elements of repeat prescribing work, including the positive role of receptionists and the value of informal over formal communication (Finn and Waring 2006) in the coordination of this work. Healthcare organisational research has focused mainly on the role of clinicians and the boundary between doctors and nurses (e.g. Allen 1997) or between clinicians and managers (e.g. Grant *et al.* 2015). With the exception of Swinglehurst *et al.* (2011), few studies have examined the role of receptionists in relation to the wider healthcare team in detail and on the role of context in augmenting this role. Given the central role of administrative team members in the quality and safety of healthcare delivery evidenced in this chapter, further research is required on the role of administrative staff within clinical contexts and on the nature of the clinical-administrative boundary as an addition to extant research on professional roles within organisational sociology.

The application of ethnographic methods has enabled us to 'exnovate' (Mesman 2012) the 'practical wisdom' and 'conjectural knowledge' (The Health Foundation 2014) employed by GPs and receptionists to conduct high-volume, everyday routine work safely and effectively. Further ethnographic studies are also required that employ the analytical lens of articulation work in order to better understand how safety and risk are understood in context. Alongside this, the study of informal, invisible safety practices can also form the basis of further 'exnovative' safety improvement work that employs ethnography and improvement methodologies such as video-reflexivity (Iedema *et al.* 2014) to foster further innovation and improvement from within healthcare organisations in order for healthcare teams themselves to better understand and build on their vulnerabilities and their strengths.

Acknowledgements

Suzanne Grant would like to thank all eight practices who generously gave up their time to participate in this study and from whom she learned so much. The authors also wish to thanks the editors and three anonymous reviewers for their constructive and insightful comments and suggestions, which greatly contributed to improving earlier versions of the manuscript. Suzanne Grant was funded by a Medical Research Council (MRC) Population Health Scientist Fellowship Award (G0802406).

References

Allen, D.A. (1997) The nursing-medical boundary: a negotiated order? *Sociology of Health & Illness*, 19, 4, 498–520.

Allen, D.A. (2014) *The Invisible Work of Nurses: Hospitals, Organisation and Healthcare.* New York: Routledge.

Arber, S. and Sawyer, L. (1985) The role of the receptionist in general practice: a 'dragon behind the desk'?, *Social Science and Medicine*, 20, 9, 911–21.

Audit Commission (1994) *A Prescription for Improvement: Towards More Rational Prescribing in General Practice.* London: Stationery Office.

Avery, T. (2010) Avoidable prescribing errors: incidence and the causes, *Prescriber*, 21, 1, 52–5.

Avery, A.J., Ghaleb, M., Barber, N., Dean Franklin, B., Armstrong, S.J., Serumaga, B., Dhillon, S., Freyer, A., Howard, R., Talabi, O. and Mehta, R.L. (2013) The prevalence and nature of prescribing and monitoring errors in UK general practice – a retrospective case note review, *British Journal of General Practice*, 63, 613, 543–53.

Bardram, J.E. (2000) Temporal coordination of time and coordination of collaborative activities at a surgical department, *Computer Supported Cooperative Work*, 9, 2, 157–87.

Bardram, J.E. and Bossen, C. (2005) Mobility work: the spatial dimension of collaboration in a hospital, *Computer Supported Cooperative Work*, 14, 2, 131–60.

Carroll, K. (2009) Unpredictable predictables: complexity theory and the construction of order in intensive care. PhD dissertation, University of Technology, Sydney (UTS)

Copeman, J. and van Zwanenberg, T. (1988) Practice receptionists: poorly paid and taken for granted? *Journal of the Royal College of General Practitioners*, 38, 1, 14–16.

Finn, R. and Waring, J. (2006) Organisational barriers to architectural knowledge and teamwork in the operating theatre, *Public Money and Management*, 26, 2, 117–24.

Fjuk, A., Smørdal, O. and Nurminen, M. (1997) Taking articulation work seriously – an activity theoretical approach. Unpublished paper submitted to ECSCW '97, Department of Informatics, University of Oslo.

Garfield, S., Barber, N., Walley, P., Willson, A. and Eliasson, L. (2009) Quality of medication use in primary care – mapping the problem, working to a solution: a systematic review of the literature, *BMC Medicine*, 7, 50.

Gherardi, S. (2006) *Organizational Knowledge. The Texture of Workplace Learning.* Oxford: Blackwell.

Grant, S., Guthrie, B., Entwistle, V.A. and Williams, B. (2014) A meta-ethnography of organisational culture in primary care medical practice, *Journal of Health Organization and Management*, 28, 1, 28–40.

Grant, S., Ring, A., Gabbay, M., Guthrie, B., McLean, G., Mair, F., Watt, G., Heaney, D. and O'Donnell, C. (2015) Soft governance, restratification and the 2004 general medical services contract: the case of UK primary care organisations and general practice teams, *Sociology of Health & Illness*, 37, 1, 30–51

Grol, R., Berwick, D. and Wensing, M. (2008) On the trail of quality and safety in health care, *British Medical Journal*, 336, 1, 74–6.

Hammond, J., Gravenhorst, K., Funnell, E., Beatty, S., Hibbert, D., Lamb, J., Burroughs, H., Kovandzic, M., Gabbay, M., Dowrick, C., Gask, L., Waheed, W. and Chew-Graham, C.A. (2013) Slaying the dragon myth: an ethnographic study of receptionists in UK general practice, *British Journal of General Practice*, 63, 608, e177–84.

Hampson, I. and Junor, A. (2005) Invisible work, invisible skills: interactive customer service as articulation work, *New Technology, Work and Employment*, 20, 2, 166–81.

Hewitt, H., McCloughan, L. and McKinstry, B. (2009) Front desk talk: discourse analysis of receptionist–patient interaction, *British Journal of General Practice*, 59, 565, 260–6.

Iedema, R. (2009) New approaches to researching patient safety, *Social Science and Medicine*, 69, 12, 1701–4.

Iedema, R., Long, D., Carroll, K., Stenglin, M. and Braithwaite, J. (2006) Corridor work: how liminal space becomes a resource for handling complexities of multi-disciplinary health care, Pacific Researchers in Organizational Studies 11th International Colloquium, 238–47. http://search. informit.com.au/documentSummary;dn=305691933675194;res=IELBUS, Accessed 27th July 2015.

Iedema, R., Mesman, J. and Carroll, K. (2014) *Visualising Healthcare Practice Improvement: Innovation from Within.* London: Radcliffe Publishing.

Law, J. (1994) *Organizing Modernity.* Oxford: Blackwell.

Macrae, C. (2014) *Close Calls: Managing Risk and Resilience in Airline Flight Safety.* Basingstoke: Palgrave.

Mays, N. and Pope, C. (1995) Rigour in qualitative research, *British Medical Journal*, 311, 6997, 109–12.

Mesman, J. (2009) The geography of patient safety: A topical analysis of sterility, *Social Science and Medicine*, 69, 12, 1705–12.

Mesman, J. (2010) Diagnostic work in collaborative practices in neonatal care. In Büscher, M., Goodwin, D. and Mesman, J. (eds) *Ethnographies of Diagnostic Work: Dimensions of Transformative Practice.* Basingstoke: Palgrave Macmillan.

Mesman, J. (2011) Resources of strength: An exnovation of hidden competences to preserve patient safety. In Rowley, E. and Waring, J. (eds) *A Socio-cultural Perspective on Patient Safety.* Aldershot: Ashgate.

Nicolini, D. (2012) *Practice Theory, Work and Organization: An Introduction.* Oxford: Oxford University Press.

Owen, C., Béguin, P. and Wackers, G. (2009) *Risky Work Environments: Reappraising Human Work within Fallible Systems.* Aldershot: Ashgate.

Petty, R., Zermansky, A.G. and Alldred, D.P. (2014) The scale of repeat prescribing – time for an update, *BMC Health Services Research*, 14, 76.

Postma, J., Oldenhof, L. and Putters, K. (2014) Organized professionalism in healthcare: articulation work by neighbourhood nurses, *Journal of Professions and Organization*, 2, 1, 61–77.

Rowley, E. and Waring, J. (2011) *A Socio-cultural Perspective on Patient Safety.* Aldershot: Ashgate.

Star, S.L. (1991) Invisible work and silenced dialogues in knowledge representation. In Ericksson, I.V., Kitchenham, B.A. and Tijdens, K.J. (eds) *Women, Work and Computerization: Understanding and Overcoming Bias in Work and Education.* Amsterdam: Elsevier.

Star, S.L. and Strauss, A. (1999) Layers of silence, arenas of voice: the ecology of visible and invisible work, *Computer Supported Cooperative Work*, 8, 1, 9–30.

Strauss, A. (1985) Work and the division of labour, *The Sociological Quarterly*, 26, 1, 1–19.

Strauss, A. (1988) The articulation of project work: An organizational process, *Sociological Quarterly*, 29, 2, 163–78.

Strauss, A. (1993) *Continual Permutations of Actions.* New York: Aldine de Gruyter.

Strauss, A., Fagerhaugh, S., Suczek, B. and Wiener, C. (1997) *The Social Organization of Medical Work.* Chicago, IL: University of Chicago Press.

Suchman, L. (1987) *Plans and Situated Action: The Problem of Human-Machine Communication.* Cambridge: Cambridge University Press.

Suchman, L. (2000) Making a case: knowledge and routine work in document production. In Luff, P., Hindmarsh, J. and Heath, C. (eds) *Workplace Studies: Recovering Work Practice and Informing System Design.* Cambridge: Cambridge University Press.

Swinglehurst, D., Greenhalgh, T., Russell, J. and Myall, M. (2011) Receptionist input to quality and safety in repeat prescribing in UK general practice: ethnographic case study, *British Medical Journal*, 343, d6788.

Taylor, R.J. (1996) Repeat prescribing – still our Achilles' heel?, *British Journal of General Practice*, 46, 412, 639–40.

The Health Foundation (2014) *Perspectives on Context: A Selection of Essays Considering the Role of Context in Successful Quality Improvement.* London: The Health Foundation.

Timmermans, S. and Freidin, B. (2007) Caretaking as articulation work: the effects of taking up responsibility for a child with asthma on labor force participation, *Social Science and Medicine*, 65, 7, 1351–63.

Ward, J. and McMurray, R. (2011) The unspoken work of GP receptionists: a re-examination of emotion management in primary care, *Social Science and Medicine*, 72, 10, 1583–7.

9

Infections and interaction rituals in the organisation: clinician accounts of speaking up or remaining silent in the face of threats to patient safety
Julia E. Szymczak

Introduction

This chapter provides a sociological examination of a behaviour that has been promoted as a technique to improve patient safety: clinicians 'speaking up' to each other and intervening in situations that might lead to harm. It is difficult for clinicians to speak up when they observe a lapse in practice. Research investigating the factors that influence speaking up typically identifies them at the individual-cognitive or on the abstract-organisational level. These explanations cannot fully account for the difficulty of speaking up because they ignore the interaction context in which healthcare is delivered.

To provide a more sophisticated and distinctly sociological understanding of this phenomenon I take seriously Collins's (1981, 2000) exhortation to place the interaction context at the centre of analysis. I use his theory of interaction ritual chains (Collins 2004) as a sensitising framework to interpret interview data in which clinicians provide accounts of their own experiences of speaking up or not when they have observed a breach in practice. The analysis shows how, through accounts given to justify speaking up or remaining silent, clinicians appeal to socially acceptable microsituational and organisational realities of medical work that shape action. These accounts demonstrate three situation-level factors that may influence the decision to speak up and illustrate how background conditions in the organisation facilitate or constrain them.

This chapter focuses on lapses in practice known to prevent the transmission of hospital-acquired infections (HAIs). HAIs are a common complication of hospital care and cause significant morbidity, mortality, excess cost and unnecessary suffering (Frieden 2010). However, they can largely be prevented by reliably taking basic precautions like handwashing (Sandora and Goldmann 2012). Reliable adherence by clinicians to basic infection prevention techniques remains a challenge for many healthcare organisations (Marra and Edmond 2012) and the act of clinicians speaking up to each other has been promoted as a technique to improve adherence (Okuyama *et al.* 2014). Unfortunately, clinicians are especially reluctant to speak up when they observe their colleagues breaching infection prevention practices (Schwappach and Gehring 2014).

'Silence kills' (Maxfield et al. 2005): speaking up and the patient safety movement
Of the factors that contribute to error in hospitals, clinician silence in the face of known threats to patient safety has been singled out as particularly disturbing and pervasive

The Sociology of Healthcare Safety and Quality, First Edition. Edited by Davina Allen, Jeffrey Braithwaite, Jane Sandall and Justin Waring. Chapters © 2016 The Authors. Book Compilation © 2016 Foundation for the Sociology of Health & Illness/Blackwell Publishing Ltd.

(Henriksen and Dayton 2006). The minimisation of patient harm via speaking up has manifested in different ways in the patient safety movement in the United States and United Kingdom over the past few decades. The creation of incident reporting systems (Lindsay *et al.* 2012) and the support of whistle-blowers who uncover incompetence and misconduct (Ehrich 2006) are two ways in which patient safety reformers have suggested silence can be overcome.

Both error reporting and whistleblowing focus on speaking up that occurs after an error happens. A third type of clinician voicing behaviour targeted by patient safety reforms is speaking up before harm reaches a patient. Analyses of safety events suggest that individuals frequently knew something was amiss but hesitated to say anything (Sutcliffe *et al.* 2004). This kind of speaking up can be defined as 'assertive communication in clinical situations that require (immediate) action through questions or statements of opinion or information with appropriate persistence until there is a clear resolution to prevent error or harm from reaching the patient' (Schwappach and Gehring 2014: 2). US hospitals have adopted practices from industries like aviation (Leonard *et al.* 2004) to encourage assertive communication. Techniques like scripted communication using 'safe words' (Sutker 2008) have been embraced by many organisations but the evidence for their impact on patient outcomes is minimal (Okuyama *et al.* 2014).

Factors that influence speaking up: the need for a relational approach
Clinicians from all professional groups have difficulty speaking up when they observe a safety threat (Maxfield *et al.* 2010). Many studies document their reluctance to verbally intervene when they witness a colleague ignoring established safety protocols (Maxfield *et al.* 2005), selecting the wrong therapy (Blatt *et al.* 2006), or neglecting to recognise or act upon a dangerous change in a patient's condition (Lyndon 2008, Simpson and Lyndon 2009). Clinicians are especially likely to remain silent when they observe their colleagues breaching infection prevention practices, such as handwashing (Samuel *et al.* 2012), appropriate glove use (Maxfield *et al.* 2010), and adherence to isolation precautions (Schwappach and Gehring 2014).

Numerous factors, typically conceptualised at either the individual-cognitive or abstract-organisational levels, have been identified to explain why clinicians are reluctant to speak up. Individual-cognitive level factors include confidence in one's knowledge of the clinical situation (Attree 2007); fear of reputational harm (Kobayashi *et al.* 2006); perception of the effectiveness of speaking up (Rutherford *et al.* 2012); perception of level of harm to the patient from the safety threat (Lyndon *et al.* 2012) and communication skills, such as ability to speak assertively (Maxfield *et al.* 2010). Identified organisational-level factors include hierarchy (Walton 2006) and status differentials (O'Connor *et al.* 2013); visible administrative support for speaking up (Edmondson 2003) and level of resources that exacerbate or mitigate clinician work stress and fatigue (Simpson and Lyndon 2009).

While these factors are useful in understanding clinician reluctance to speak up, they cannot fully account for this phenomenon because they do not capture the nuances of people interacting with each other in time and space. These factors as currently conceptualised leave the possible mechanisms that influence speaking up under-specified. Clinical scholars working in this area suggest a greater empirical emphasis on the fluid nature of communication in healthcare. Espin *et al.* (2006: 170) suggest that individual-cognitive and organisational explanations for the difficulty of speaking up are unable 'to fully account for the role of human social relationships in the everyday persistence of unsafe practice' and neglect 'the dimension of interaction that lies between [individuals and organisations] – the everyday human contact and social formation of friendships and conflicts that occur when individuals work in groups'. Blatt *et al.* (2006) suggest that we need to move beyond explanations that emphasise personality differences or organisational climate and instead consider the influence of the 'relational environment', or those factors that arise out of the relationships between people at particular points in time.

Using microsociological theory to connect the interaction context with the organisational level

To advance our understanding of the challenges of speaking up in clinical settings we need to further explore the role of the interaction context. This is where a distinctly sociological approach to patient safety, as opposed to focusing only on individual psychology or abstract macro concepts such as 'hierarchy' or 'culture', can be of great value. In a sociological approach, the interaction itself is examined to develop a more sophisticated understanding of the way clinicians navigate opportunities to speak up to prevent patient harm. I draw on the work of Collins (1981, 1988, 2000, 2004), who has long suggested that sociologists can advance explanatory theories by building connections between the microrealities of everyday experience and macrosociological phenomena. Microsociological theory can assist us by drawing our analytic attention to practical, face-to-face encounters.

In this chapter, I use Collins's (2004) theory of interaction ritual chains (IRCs) as an analytic framework. This general theoretical model combines Durkheim's (1912) emphasis on solidarity as it is produced in rituals via collective effervescence with Goffman's (1967) microsociological emphasis on face-to-face interaction. It posits that face-to-face interaction rituals (IRs) are the main mechanism that holds society together. There are four key ingredients to an IR that, if successfully combined, build up high levels of emotional entrainment, resulting in favourable outcomes that perpetuate more IRs: (i) physical co-presence; (ii) barriers to outsiders; (iii) mutual focus of attention; and (iv) shared mood. Outcomes of the combination of these four ingredients include: (i) group solidarity; (ii) emotional energy in the individual; (iii) symbols that represent the group; and (iv) feelings of morality (Collins 2004: 48–9).

An elaboration of one of these ritual outcome variables – emotional energy – will be useful to analysis in this case. Emotional energy (EE) is an integral part of the IRC model and contributes greatly to our understanding of human motivation. In IRC theory, an individual's level of EE is the long-term emotional outcome that results from IRs. It is expressed along a continuum from high (confidence, enthusiasm) to low (depression, negative feeling). The desire for EE catalyses people to take initiative and engage in social action. Individuals either gain or lose EE depending on the nature of the interaction.

A second aspect of IRC theory that is useful to this case is the idea that people's lives are made up of 'chains' of IRs. Individuals encounter a variety of situations that could involve an IR. How they navigate these situations forms the basis of a market for IRs. The key to this market is that people are EE seekers; they gravitate to situations in which their EE payoff will be highest. In the IR chain model, people move from situation to situation, choosing to engage in some IRs but not others based on how each 'participant's stock of social resources – their EE and membership symbols accumulated in previous IRs – meshes with those of each person they encounter' (Collins 2004: xiv). People leave an IR having their social resources bolstered or depleted and continue on to new IRs, each time having these two interactional resources altered.

By thinking about clinicians speaking up to each other about breaches in practice as a type of IR, I seek to not only describe the possible microdynamics of speaking up, but also to connect them with features of organisational life that facilitate or constrain them. While Collins (1988, 2000) is a proponent of microsociology, he suggests that the examination of core sociological concepts like stratification is most fruitfully accomplished by moving between levels of analysis.

Accessing interactions through accounts: narrating situational and
organisational realities

Ideally, to study speaking up in clinical settings as a microsociological phenomenon, one would gather detailed ethnographic data supplemented with audio-visual recordings to capture the dynamics of face-to-face interaction *in situ*. While this approach is preferable to qualitative interviewing, it is not a perfect solution in that it is likely difficult to observe from afar (in the case of video recorded interactions) the factors that shape the decision to speak up or not, especially as they manifest in the mind of an individual (Collins 2004). Additionally, the presence of an observer could impact the unfolding action in ways that might influence the dynamics of the microsituation under study.

Interviews can provide useful insight about a phenomenon of interest as long as we treat them as interactional events and recognise that verbal accounts produced by respondents are a form of action aimed at social signalling (Khan and Jerolmack 2013). In the research interview a respondent works to portray himself or herself as a credible person (Holstein and Gubrium 1995). Interviews thus have a storied form. The stories told in interviews can be systematically analysed to identify the work they do to appeal to features of a social world that render the respondent's behaviour acceptable. These appeals exhibit a set of socially accepted rationales for action or inaction that, when laid bare, give us a deeper understanding of a particular phenomenon. In this chapter I provide an analysis of verbal accounts generated in interviews with clinicians wherein they reflect on past experience speaking up or not when they observed a breach in infection prevention practice. I treat these accounts as stories of interactional microsituations that are produced by clinicians to communicate something meaningful to a sociologist.

The analysis of accounts given by individuals to explain their conduct and to bolster their claim to legitimacy has a long history in sociology (Mills 1940, Scott and Lyman 1968). This literature exhorts scholars to take seriously the verbal statements made by people when their behaviour falls short of societal expectations. As Scott and Lyman (1968: 61) suggest 'we want to know how… actors take bits and pieces of words and appearances and put them together to produce a perceived normal (or abnormal) state of affairs'. Accounts can be understood as ways that people 'neutralise' deviant behaviour (Sykes and Matza 1957) by managing culpability, make meaning about a particular life experience (Allen 2012) and establish their identity (Scott and Lyman 1968). In medical sociology, scholars have used the concept of accounts to examine topics such as infant feeding (Murphy 1999), steroid use among bodybuilders (Monaghan 2002) and the way mothers parent adolescents living with diabetes (Allen 2012).

Beyond the neutralisation and identity work that accounts do, they also provide important insight into the social world in which the individual giving the account is enmeshed (Allen 2012). For example, Baruch (1981: 282, my emphasis), in examining parents' stories of encounters with doctors in which they justify their delay in seeking care for their seriously ill children, argues that when individuals accomplish moral displays through accounts 'they appeal *to features of their world and show how according to these features they acted reasonably, consistently and competently* given the situations described in their stories'. Accounts can be examined as forms of justification that communicate features of an actor's social reality that render the behaviour comprehensible. It is this aspect of account giving that I focus on in this chapter.

In what follows, I apply an analytic lens informed by IRC theory to the interpretation of accounts given by clinicians of interactional microsituations to justify speaking up or remaining silent. My aim is to identify the situational and organisational realities that are communicated through these accounts in order to develop a more sophisticated understanding of the social dynamics of communication challenges in healthcare.

Methods

Data collection
The data for this chapter were gathered in the context of a 2-year (2010–2012) ethnographic study investigating the implementation of an infection prevention campaign at a paediatric hospital (referred to pseudonymously as 'Stonegate') in the US. I primarily observed infection prevention practitioners, a group of healthcare workers who do not provide hands-on clinical care. Rather their job is to educate, audit behaviour, develop policies and identify infections as hospital-acquired. The secondary focus of my observations was meetings of Stonegate's 'Prevent Infection' campaign. This hospital-wide campaign was focused on reducing HAIs via implementation of various patient safety strategies, described elsewhere (Szymczak 2014). I did not observe frontline clinicians as they provided patient care due to access restrictions.

The analyses presented here are based upon semistructured, in-depth interviews conducted with a purposive sample of 103 Stonegate staff, of which 75 were frontline clinicians (doctors, nurses and respiratory therapists). My sample included staff that varied on three axes: occupational group, organisational strata and primary work area (Table 1). The overall response rate was 88.79 per cent and I recruited respondents until I reached thematic saturation. All interviews were conducted in person, recorded and lasted from 45 minutes to 4 hours, with an average time of 86 minutes. The Institutional Review Board approved this study. Informed consent was obtained from all participants.

My interview guide included a subset of questions about speaking up upon observing a breach in practice because this emerged as a formal organisational goal of Stonegate's 'Prevent Infection' campaign. Hospital leadership believed that they could reduce rates of infection if they could get staff to speak up to stop breaches. Leaders attempted to implement various improvement activities such as teaching scripted communication to use upon confronting a breach. Consistent with the literature reviewed above, Stonegate clinicians struggled to speak up. The questions in my interview guide about speaking up were designed to elicit accounts justifying action or inaction that included micro-level detail. I wanted to understand what it was like to be in this situation and to probe for accounts

Table 1   *Characteristics of interview sample (n = 103)*

	n
Occupational group	
Nurse	56
Physician	30
Respiratory therapist	5
Other	12
Organisational strata	
Top leader	18
Mid-level manager	10
Frontline clinical staff	75
Primary work location	
ICU	39
OR	18
General paediatrics ward	14
Other specialty	14
Patient safety department	18

that moved beyond the usual explanations given by administrators about the difficulties of speaking up – 'it's the hierarchy' or that people were not 'brave enough' to voice concerns.

I started by asking my respondents how comfortable they were speaking up about breaches in infection prevention practice. Then, I asked if they could explain in detail an occasion where they spoke up, the situation surrounding the breach and how the resulting interaction went. I probed for details about the clinical situation, the respondents' emotional feeling, what thoughts ran through their minds, the physical environment, what they said and how the people they spoke to responded. Following this, I asked whether they could recall the opposite situation – a time when they observed breaches in practice but did not speak up – and to recount the same details.

Analysis
All interviews were transcribed verbatim and uploaded to NVivo 10 (QSR International, Brisbane) qualitative data analysis software for thematic coding. I read through all documents line-by-line in a process of open coding, creating theme categories or 'nodes' that were attached to passages of data that could later be sorted and further analysed. During open coding, I created a node called 'speaking up' that captured all discussions of assertive communication by clinicians to stop breaches in practice. I isolated this node and performed a more focused analysis of these accounts, using the ingredients-outcomes model of IRC theory to understand the work that these accounts do to make speaking up or remaining silent appear reasonable and credible given the social world of medical work.

Results

Finding mutual focus of attention in a complex, time-pressured clinical work setting
In their accounts, clinicians frequently gave detailed descriptions of the pace, 'feel' and physical reality of providing patient care in a highly complex, time-pressured clinical work setting as part of their justifications for speaking up or remaining silent. The first situation-level factor that clinicians appealed to in their accounts is having a mutual focus of attention. To have a successful IR, participants must be physically co-present, focus their attention upon a common object or activity and be aware of the object of their shared focus (Collins 2004). This results in a high level of entrainment that facilitates the interaction. My respondents communicated to me the reality that, although they may be sharing close physical space with colleagues, they may not be focusing on the same thing:

> We should be speaking up about hub scrubs [a central line infection prevention practice], but sometimes you just aren't on the same page even if you work closely together. Yesterday I was involved in a crazy task – my patient was trying to sit up with his breathing tube in and I'm suctioning, trying to keep him calm, and a nurse was next to me preparing to push a [routine] med through the central line and she is literally standing right next to me, we're almost touching, but I didn't notice whether she scrubbed the hub because I'm concentrating on my own thing. (Nurse, Intensive Care Unit [ICU])

In this account, the respondent vividly describes the complicated nature of clinical labour to communicate that, despite being in very close physical proximity to one another, workers in busy clinical settings may not share a mutual focus of attention, which justifies silence.

This reflects an organisational reality facing virtually all hospitals in the US: clinicians are expected to care for more patients with more complex medical needs and to discharge them faster than ever before (Edmond 2010). Hospital administrators focus on increasing the efficiency of their workforce with the consequence that clinicians end up performing multiple tasks at the same time in such a way that constrains them from having a mutual focus of attention. During my fieldwork, Stonegate's administration had begun a clinical productivity initiative aimed at improving nurse efficiency. In my observations, this emerged as a competing organisational priority that threatened nurses' ability to fully embrace strategies to prevent infection.

Contrast the first account with the following, in which the respondent describes how a group of clinicians having a mutual focus of attention facilitated speaking up:

> I was working as part of a multidisciplinary team in a very complex moment in the NICU [neonatal intensive care unit] – putting a baby on ECMO [extra-corporeal membrane oxygenation] and I spoke up to another physician about hand hygiene. I just said 'here's the gel' as they were about to put on gloves. It felt like we were a well-oiled machine, circling the bedside tightly – working together to achieve one goal – to put the child on ECMO. We'd done a time out, we knew each other's names, we were all focused on the same thing. (Physician, NICU)

This account has a very different tenor than the previous one. Although the task described is arguably more medically complex (putting a baby on ECMO versus pushing routine medications through a central line), the clinical team had in place all of the main ingredients necessary for a successful IR – group assembly, a barrier to outsides ('circling the bedside tightly'), a mutual focus of attention on one task and shared mood facilitated by the time out. This is a safety technique used prior to invasive procedures to assure, among other things, that the procedure is being performed on the correct patient and body site. Stonegate had formalised organisational protocols mandating that clinicians have a time out for certain procedures, like ECMO. As communicated through this account, a time out also serves an interactional function that can promote assertive communication – it forces a pause in the action that encourages a mutual focus of attention. This facilitates speaking up because individuals are highly entrained with each other.

Through their accounts, my respondents described how giving feedback when there is no mutual focus of attention is not only difficult, but also entails interactional risks that may be more dangerous to the patient than the risk of infection:

> You have to be careful when you speak up, timing-wise, in our area. If you see someone breaching an infection prevention practice from across the room you really have to think about whatever else is going on at that moment. So do you want to say, 'you just broke sterility' when the doctor has his hands in a chest or is holding onto a cardiac catheter in a groin? No, you just don't do that because what if the person gets angry, erupts at you, then what? That would be very risky for the patient – more risky than an infection in that moment. (Nurse, Operating Room)

By including a question posed to the interviewer in her account, this nurse urgently appeals to the kind of moment-to-moment competing priorities that frontline clinicians must navigate on a daily basis. In situations where a colleague is concentrating on a task and the person speaking up is peripheral to that task, my respondents justified remaining silent because of the possibility that speaking up might provoke volatile emotional reactions.

In their accounts, respondents used patterned phrases like 'lash out', 'have a meltdown', 'explode', 'blast off',and 'unravel' to justify remaining silent at times when speaking up was likely to be so jarring to the person being spoken to that their response would be detrimental to safety. When the 'frame' that specifies assumptions about what is going on at a particular moment is broken an intense emotional response, 'flooding out', can occur (Goffman 1974). Especially in moments where a clinician's body is engaged in care that requires a delicate touch, the interactional risk of 'flooding out' emotion has the potential to contribute to error by overwhelming bodily control. Clinicians not only consider the possible harm to the patient that a particular breach in practice represents (Lyndon *et al.* 2012), they also consider the harm that may occur to the patient as a result of the interactional conditions of the situation if they do speak up.

Path dependence: the importance of past interactions
The second situational factor that clinicians appealed to in their accounts is a consideration of past interactions. When justifying speaking up or remaining silent, clinicians frequently described that the choice they made in any one moment was shaped by past interactions, even if far removed from or unrelated to the observed breach. In other words, speaking up is inter-actionally path dependent. Path dependence describes how the set of decisions one faces for any given circumstance is mediated by the decisions one has made in the past, even though past circumstances may no longer be immediately relevant (Sewell 1996). Per IRC theory, our lives are made up of 'chains' of IRs. Our propensity to engage in an IR is tempered by the level of EE and stock of membership symbols we have accumulated in past IRs. In their accounts of speaking up, respondents described how past interactions shaped their decision to intervene:

> You have many points of care to get through each day. You have many battles to fight with multiple disciplines and that gets exhausting so you learn to pick your battles. Sometimes you're tired, you've already had three fights with a person, they're in a cranky mood ... and arguing over a stupid yellow [isolation] gown is just the last thing on your mind ... You've already had many arguments with this person on patient care, on critical issues.

> And it's not that infections aren't critical, but the odds of her spreading RSV [respiratory syncytial virus] when she barely touches a patient while not wearing a yellow gown are slim to none, so that is how I decide whether it is worth it to say anything or not. (Physician, ICU)

This physician justifies remaining silent in the face of a hypothetical but common-in-practice breach by communicating the situational reality that fatigue from previous strained interac-tions with a colleague, plus her own doubt about the risk that would arise from the breach in practice, come together to shape behaviour. Her account utilises a sentence that strings together past events and background conditions ('Sometimes you're tired ...') to vividly jus-tify why speaking up does not occur. Conversely, clinicians also described how positive past interactions can facilitate speaking up:

> Once I gave feedback to a doctor who was examining a baby with a whole team. His tie was dangling in the bed and he kept touching his glasses. I stopped him and was polite. I said, 'excuse me'. And I explained to him what I saw. He was extremely grateful and thanked me profusely in front of everyone. That felt really good – I felt proud. He told other people about it because our Director of Nursing found me to thank me for speaking up for patient safety ... It made me feel so empowered to speak up again, which I now do all the time. (Nurse, NICU)

This nurse provides an account of how she felt after giving feedback that was well-received. Interpreted through the lens of IRC theory, the nurse is describing an EE-bolstering interaction, the energy and positive feeling from which reverberated, serving as a catalyst for her to engage in more interactions. In this situation, the organisation's emphasis on speaking up as a behaviour to be lauded served to amplify the effects of this IR. Stonegate leaders emphasised the importance of telling stories publicly of situations when clinicians spoke up to successfully stop a breach in practice. It was a formal organisational practice to start each meeting of the 'Prevent Infection' initiative with a 'safety story', the majority of which centred on clinicians speaking up to each other to stop a breach in practice.

The importance of past interactions was further elaborated in many of my respondent's accounts when they justified speaking up to individuals whom they knew and had many intense interactions with in the past:

> Recently one of our senior cardiothoracic surgeons was coming into my patient's room to examine the surgical wound and I saw him go towards the dressing without doing hand hygiene and I stepped closer to him and said, 'Stop. Wash your hands before you touch that, come on!' And he thanked me. But I felt like I could do that because we have recently been through a lot together, we've been through many critical times in the middle of the night with sick patients, very intense and emotional situations where we worked together well. We had shared history so I felt I could say something. (Nurse, ICU)

Here, a relatively junior nurse (2 years out of training) justifies speaking up to a senior surgeon because of the positive emotional reverberations from past interactions. She utilises the word 'we' throughout the account to highlight their shared history. This account complicates a reason that is typically given for why speaking up in clinical settings is so difficult: hierarchy. As Collins (2000) suggests, our abstract macro conceptualisations of 'hierarchy' and 'inequality' frequently do not come to grips with the reality of lived experience. By investigating the situational experience of stratification we can identify possible micromechanisms that account for cases that do not fit our current explanations. This nurse's account points to the role of past interactions in shaping a clinician's propensity to speak up and transcend the limits of hierarchy as we traditionally think about it in medical work settings.

Whether an individual will have had successful past IRs with an individual that can facilitate speaking up at any one moment is shaped by organisational conditions. Organisational change and its impact on opportunities for individuals to build up chains of interactions can be observed in the following account from an emergency room (ER) physician who justifies not speaking up to a nurse who had a breach in hand hygiene by appealing to a consequence of hospital growth – people do not know each other's names:

> The other day I was charting outside a patient's room and saw a nurse not wash her hands before going to touch the kid and I didn't say anything to her because, honestly, I didn't know her name and I couldn't see her [identification] badge. So 10 years ago, you know, Stonegate was smaller. I would have told you that I knew every single ER nurse here; that I had shared overnights with them. We had worked side by side in the trenches. We had been through lots of stuff together. We just knew how to dance. You know? And now, I really don't have that anymore. We've grown so much, increased our size and the number of patients the hospital expects us to see. So I don't know all the nurses. Like, maybe I know 50% of them by sight, but not their name, you know? And the hugeness of this place causes this. (Physician, ICU)

The use of a dance metaphor conveys how past interactions had a fluid, seamless, knowing quality whereas present interactions are missing this familiarity. Organisational growth can constrain the ability of clinicians to develop a chain of past successful interactions with each other that may facilitate speaking up in the future.

Presence of an audience
The final situational condition that clinicians appealed to in their accounts is that clinical work is frequently performed in front of an audience. Collins suggests that IRs are facilitated when there is a barrier to outsiders. In clinical settings, respondents communicated to me, the barrier between insiders and outsiders is permeable and in flux. A situational reality that was oft repeated in their accounts is that clinical work is frequently performed in front of audiences, including patients, families and colleagues who are constantly judging competence. Respondents described how they take into account the other people who are present in any one situation when deciding to speak up:

> I saw a senior surgeon talking to a family and leaning his hands and arms on the baby's crib. And the baby had MRSA [Methicillin-resistant *Staphylococcus aureus*]. And he wasn't wearing a gown. And in my mind I said 'take your hands off that crib, he has MRSA!' but then I said, 'well, he's talking to the family.' And I could tell it was a serious conversation, the baby was not doing well. If no family was there I would have been able to say 'oh, he is on precautions, can you put on a gown and gloves?' (Physician, NICU)

In this account, a physician recounts the self-talk that went through her mind upon witnessing a breach committed by a senior surgeon. She communicates how she could tell from subtle signals that the conversation with the parents was a serious one, which justified her remaining silent. Many of my respondents justified not speaking up at moments during everyday clinical work when parents of critically ill children were present. Great concern was expressed across respondents about controlling the impression that parents received of the clinical action unfolding in front of them (Goffman 1959). This is largely because, my respondents explained, speaking up about breaches in infection prevention was thought to threaten an individual's projection of competence.

This concern was likely influenced by a larger organisational dynamic that characterised Stonegate as a well-known paediatric hospital: in addition to providing care to critically ill children, clinicians needed to navigate parent expectations and assure satisfaction. Throughout my research I found clinicians providing accounts of interactions with parents that caused tension with the goal of preventing infection. Frontline clinical staff explained to me that they felt a lot of pressure to make parents happy. Stonegate, like many hospitals in the US, encourages parents to fill out satisfaction surveys at the conclusion of a hospitalisation. Satisfaction scores were used as one metric at the administrative level to monitor clinician performance. This organisational dynamic, coupled with the fact that parents are frequently present at the bedside of their hospitalised child, was frequently noted as a constraint on speaking up.

In justifying speaking up or remaining silent in the presence of an audience, clinicians suggested they were particularly sensitive to their colleague's need to establish credibility, not only with parents but also with clinical superiors. Stonegate is a teaching hospital and the social dynamics surrounding healthcare training that have long been a focus of medical sociology research (e.g. Becker *et al.* 1961) were omnipresent in organisational life. My respondents appealed to these dynamics in talking about how they oriented to what speaking up about a breach in practice meant for the person being spoken to. A respiratory therapist provides an account of a time she moderated the way she spoke up about a breach to a physician trainee:

I was standing behind a new anaesthesiology fellow, working with his attending to extubate a patient. He let the oral suction catheter fall to the floor. I watched him look around to see if anyone noticed. They hadn't. He picked up the tube, but before he put it back in [the patient's mouth] I said, 'here is another suction catheter'. He put his head down and said 'thank you'. I knew he was worried about delaying things, about his attending not thinking he was efficient. I also knew I couldn't make a big deal about him dropping the catheter in front of his attending. Maybe if we were alone I would have said more but I didn't want to jeopardise his relationship with the attending because he is brand new.

In this case the respiratory therapist recounts how she intervened to stop a risky practice, but justifies doing so in a subtle way that was sensitive to the social vulnerability of the trainee she spoke to. Successful IRs are more likely to occur when there is a clear delineation between those who are taking part in the interaction and those who are not. Because clinical work is performed in front of people who are constantly judging competence, the boundary between insiders and outsiders is blurred in such a way as to make it difficult for clinicians to enter an IR around breaches in practice.

Discussion

The decision to speak up or remain silent about a breach in practice at any one moment in clinical settings is dynamic, highly context-dependent and embedded in the daily interaction rituals that suffuse work in a complex organisation. This chapter investigates the challenges that clinicians have in speaking up to each other to stop threats to patient safety. My analysis is innovative in that it picks up calls from scholars including Blatt *et al.* (2006) and Espin *et al.* (2006), to focus on the relational environment and pushes their analyses in new directions by taking a distinctively sociological approach that emphasises the role of the interaction context.

By examining the appeals that clinicians make to situational and organisational realities in their accounts of speaking up or remaining silent, I have generated deeper insight into the dynamics that facilitate or constrain the process. By focusing my analytic attention on accounts of interactions between individual people, my goal has been to recouple the challenges of clinical communication to the dynamic, situated and contingent experience of people doing work together on people in a busy clinical environment nestled in a complex organisational sphere. This analysis advances our understanding of the factors that may influence the integration of patient safety-promoting behaviours, such as speaking up, in everyday work.

Accounts given by clinicians appeal to three micro-level dynamics that may influence the decision to speak up or remain silent: having a mutual focus of attention; past interactions that facilitate or stymie engaging in interactions around a breach; and the presence of an audience. These dynamics manifest at the microinteractional level but are, as the analysis shows, shaped by features of organisational life that facilitate or constrain their expression. Stonegate's task complexity, production pressures, formal safety protocols, supportive leadership, physical growth, increasing attention paid to patient satisfaction as a proxy for performance and its academic mission are all organisational level factors that shaped the situational reality of my respondent's work experiences. While past research has identified administrative support (Edmondson 2003) and work stress (Simpson and Lyndon 2009) as factors that influence speaking up, until now we did not have a sense of the possible mechanisms by which these organisational-level dynamics shape experience. Sociological theory, as opposed to research that focuses exclusively on psychological dynamics or organisational climate, allows us to identify micromechanisms that have remained under-specified.

Consistent with the findings of other sociological studies of patient safety, my study highlights the influence of social and political concerns on the integration of safety techniques (Dixon-Woods *et al.* 2009, Lindsay *et al.* 2012). Social relationships are frequently at stake in any encounter between individuals in a clinical setting. Medical reforms can have a deeper meaning to the people who are affected by them than the reform's operational impact on error (Kellogg 2011). My study reaffirms the need to consider the social risk inherent in patient safety tools and techniques. My respondents, in making the decision to speak up or not, balance one risk against another – and occasionally, the social risk emerged as more serious in any one moment than the risk of infection.

As scholars have identified, the perception of harm that will come to a patient from remaining silent is an important mediating factor influencing whether a clinician will speak up (Lyndon *et al.* 2012). This chapter has focused on the risk of HAI, a type of harm that may have a very different motivating effect than other types of patient harm. Throughout the results section we can see clinicians appealing to the need to balance the social risk of speaking up with the less-certain risk of the patient acquiring an infection from a breach in practice. Hospital-acquired infections are not as 'dramatic' as other types of medical harm, such as wrong-site surgery or a medication error leading to an overdose. Infections are less dramatic because it is almost impossible to link any given infection to the behaviour that caused it. There are also often delays in feedback in that non-compliance with an infection prevention practice does not typically have a direct and immediately observable result (Dixon-Woods *et al.* 2009). The social construction of risk perception (Douglas and Wildavsky 1982) matters fatefully for clinician voicing behaviour and should be considered in future studies of the topic.

This study, as a result of the methods used, has limitations. First, I have relied on interview data to explore the social dynamics of speaking up behaviour. As I suggest at the outset, interviews are interaction events that produce accounts of action that have a storied form and are communicated as a form of social signalling (Khan and Jerolmack 2013). There are limits to what these data can tell us about actual speaking up behaviour. The accounts that people give about their behaviour and the actual reasons that they behave the way they do may be quite different. Ethnographic observations of clinicians speaking up to each other *in situ* may provide a more complete picture of this phenomenon, although this approach is also not without its limitations. Second, this study was conducted at one hospital, so the results may not be generalisable to other clinical settings, although there is no reason to believe that the social and organisational dynamics that characterise medical work at Stonegate are radically different from other settings. Despite these limitations, a study of this type is an important first step in examining how situational and organisational realities may shape the enactment of a particular patient safety behaviour.

The choice to speak up or remain silent in a clinical setting is influenced not only by the microdynamics of individual bodies in physical space, but also the history between people and social relationships at stake in any encounter in a medical work setting. These factors are embedded within a complex organisational environment that facilitates or constrains them. In addition to identifying possible reasons why clinicians speak up or remain silent, this chapter highlights the analytic leverage that can be gained by recoupling patient safety techniques to the microdynamics of social interaction. Future research should consider the dynamics of social interaction when considering how different patient safety practices are integrated into medical work.

Acknowledgements

Funding for this project was provided by a US Agency for Healthcare Research & Quality R36 Health Services Research Dissertation Grant (1R36HS020760-01) and a University of Pennsylvania School of Arts and Sciences Graduate Division Dissertation Completion Fellowship.

References

Allen, D. (2012) 'Just a typical teenager': The social ecology of 'normal adolescence' – insights from diabetes care, *Symbolic Interaction*, 36, 1, 40–59.

Attree, M. (2007) Factors influencing nurses' decisions to raise concerns about care quality. *Journal of Nursing Management*, 15, 4, 392–402.

Baruch, G. (1981) Moral tales: Parents' stories of encounters with the health professions, *Sociology of Health and Illness*, 3, 3, 275–95.

Becker, H.S., Geer, B., Hughes, E. and Strauss, A.L. (1961) *Boys in White: Student Culture in Medical School*. Chicago, IL: University of Chicago Press.

Blatt, R., Christianson, M.K., Sutcliffe, K.M. and Rosenthal, M.M. (2006) A sensemaking lens on reliability, *Journal of Organizational Behavior*, 27, 7, 897–917.

Collins, R. (1981) On the microfoundations of macrosociology, *American Journal of Sociology*, 86, 5, 984–1014.

Collins, R. (1988) The micro contribution to macro sociology, *Sociological Theory*, 6, 2, 242–53.

Collins, R. (2000) Situational stratification: A micro-macro theory of inequality, *Sociological Theory*, 18, 1, 17–43.

Collins, R. (2004) *Interaction Ritual Chains*. Princeton, NJ: Princeton University Press.

Dixon-Woods, M., Suokas, A., Pitchforth, E. and Tarrant, C. (2009) An ethnographic study of classifying and accounting for risk at the sharp end of medical wards, *Social Science & Medicine*, 69, 3, 362–9.

Douglas, M. and Wildavsky, A. (1982) *Risk and Culture: An Essay on the Selection of Technological and Environmental Dangers*. Berkeley, CA: University of California Press.

Durkheim, E. (1912) *The Elementary Forms of Religious Life*. Translated by Fields, K.E. (1995), New York: Free Press.

Edmond, M.B. (2010) Taylorized medicine, *Annals of Internal Medicine*, 153, 12, 845–6.

Edmondson, A.C. (2003) Speaking up in the operating room: how team leaders promote learning in interdisciplinary action teams, *Journal of Management Studies*, 40, 6, 1419–52.

Ehrich, K. (2006) Telling cultures: 'Cultural' issues for staff reporting concerns about colleagues in the UK National Health Service, *Sociology of Health & Illness*, 28, 7, 903–26.

Espin, S., Lingard, L., Baker, G.R. and Regehr, G. (2006) Persistence of unsafe practice in everyday work: An exploration of organizational and psychological factors constraining safety in the operating room, *Quality and Safety in Healthcare*, 15, 3, 165–70.

Frieden, T.R. (2010) Maximizing infection prevention in the next decade: Defining the unacceptable, *Infection Control & Hospital Epidemiology*, 31, Suppl 1, 1–3.

Goffman, E. (1959) *The Presentation of Self in Everyday Life*. New York: Anchor Books Doubleday.

Goffman, E. (1967) *Interaction Ritual*. New York: Doubleday.

Goffman, E. (1974) *Frame Analysis*. Boston, MA: Northeastern University Press.

Greenberg, C.C., Regenbogen, S.E., Studdert, D.M., Lipsitz, S.R., *et al.* (2007) Patterns of communication breakdowns resulting in injury to surgical patients, *Journal of the American College of Surgery*, 204, 4, 533–40.

Henriksen, K. and Dayton, E. (2006) Organizational silence and hidden threats to patient safety, *Health Services Research*, 41, 4, 1539–54.

Holstein, J.A. and Gubrium, J.F. (1995) *The Active Interview.* Thousand Oaks, CA: Sage.

Kellogg, K.C. (2011) *Challenging Operations: Medical Reform and Resistance in Surgery.* Chicago, IL: University of Chicago Press.

Khan, S. and Jerolmack, C. (2013) Saying meritocracy and doing privilege, *The Sociological Quarterly*, 54, 1, 9–19.

Kobayashi, H., Pian-Smith, M., Sato, M., Sawa, R., *et al.* (2006) A cross-cultural survey of residents' perceived barriers in questioning/challenging authority, *Quality and Safety in Healthcare*, 15, 4, 277–83.

Leonard, M., Graham, S. and Bonacum, D. (2004) The human factor: the critical importance of effective teamwork and communication in providing safe care, *Quality and Safety in Health Care*, 13, 1, 85–90.

Lewis, G.H., Vaithianathan, R., Hockey, P.M., Hirst, G., *et al.* (2011) Counterheroism, common knowledge, and ergonomics: Concepts from aviation that could improve patient safety, *Milbank Quarterly*, 89, 1, 4–38.

Lindsay, P., Sandall, J. and Humphrey, C. (2012) The social dimensions of safety incident reporting in maternity care: The influence of working relationships and group processes, *Social Science & Medicine*, 75, 10, 1793–9.

Lyndon, A. (2008) Social and environmental conditions creating fluctuating agency for safety in two urban academic birth centers, *Journal of Obstetric, Gynecologic & Neonatal Nursing*, 37, 1, 13–23.

Lyndon, A., Sexton, J.B., Simpson, K.R., Rosenstein, A., *et al.* (2012) Predictors of likelihood of speaking up about safety concerns in labour and delivery, *BMJ Quality and Safety*, 21, 9, 791–9.

Marra, A.R. and Edmond, M.B. (2012) Hand hygiene: State-of-the-art review with emphasis on new technologies and mechanisms of surveillance, *Current Infectious Disease Report*, 14, 6, 585–91.

Maxfield, D., Grenny, J., McMillan, R., Patterson, K., *et al.* (2005) Silence kills. Available at http://www.aacn.org/WD/practice/docs/publicpolicy/silencekills.pdf. Date last accessed 28 July 2014.

Maxfield, D., Grenny, J., Lavandero, R. and Groah, L. (2010) The silent treatment. Available at http://www.aacn.org/WD/hwe/docs/the-silent-treatment.pdf. Date last accessed 28 July 2014.

Mills, C.W. (1940) Situated actions and vocabularies of motive, *American Sociological Review*, 5, 6, 904–13.

Monaghan, L.F. (2002) Vocabularies of motive for illicit steroid use among bodybuilders, *Social Science and Medicine*, 55, 5, 695–708.

Murphy, E. (1999) 'Breast is best': Infant feeding decisions and maternal deviance, *Sociology of Health & Illness*, 21, 2, 187–208.

O'Connor, P., Byrne, D., O'Dea, A., McVeigh, T.P., *et al.* (2013) 'Excuse Me:' Teaching interns to speak up, *The Joint Commission Journal on Quality and Patient Safety*, 39, 9, 426–31.

Okuyama, A., Wagner, C. and Bijnen, B. (2014) Speaking up for patient safety by hospital-based healthcare professionals: A literature review, *BMC Health Services Research*, 14, 61.

Rutherford, J.S., Flin, R. and Mitchell, L. (2012) Teamwork, communication, and anaesthetic assistance in Scotland, *British Journal of Anesthesia*, 109, 1, 21–6.

Samuel, R., Shuen, A., Dendle, C., Kotsanas, D., *et al.* (2012) Hierarchy and hand hygiene: would medical students speak up to prevent hospital-acquired infection? *Infection Control & Hospital Epidemiology*, 33, 8, 861–3.

Sandora, T.J. and Goldmann, D.A. (2012) Preventing lethal hospital outbreaks of antibiotic-resistant bacteria, *New England Journal of Medicine*, 367, 23, 2168–70.

Schwappach, D.L.B. and Gehring, K. (2014) 'Saying it without words': a qualitative study of oncology staff's experiences with speaking up about safety concerns, *BMJ Open*, 4, e004740.

Scott, M.B. and Lyman, S.M. (1968) Accounts, *American Sociological Review*, 33, 1, 46–62.

Sewell, W.H. (1996) Three temporalities: Toward an eventful sociology. In McDonald, T.J. (ed) *The Historic Turn in the Human Sciences.* Ann Arbor, MI: University of Michigan Press.

Simpson, K.R. and Lyndon, A. (2009) Clinical disagreements during labor and birth: How does real life compare to best practice? *The American Journal of Maternal/Child Nursing*, 34, 1, 31–9.

Sutcliffe, K.M., Lewton, E. and Rosenthal, M.M. (2004) Communication failures: An insidious contributor to medical mishaps, *Academic Medicine*, 79, 2, 189–94.

Sutker, W.L. (2008) The physician's role in patient safety: what's in it for me?, *Baylor University Medical Center Proceedings*, 21, 1, 9–14.

Sykes, D.M. and Matza, D. (1957) Techniques of neutralization: A theory of delinquency, *American Sociological Review*, 22, 6, 664–70.

Szymczak, J.E. (2014) Seeing risk and allocating responsibility: Talk of culture and its consequences on the work of patient safety, *Social Science and Medicine*, 120, 252–9.

Walton, M.M. (2006) Hierarchies: The Berlin Wall of patient safety, *Quality and Safety in Healthcare*, 15, 4, 229–30.

Index

Page numbers in **bold** indicate tables; page numbers in *italics* indicate figures.

The Sociology of Healthcare Safety and Quality, First Edition. Edited by Davina Allen, Jeffrey Braithwaite,
Jane Sandall and Justin Waring. Chapters © 2016 The Authors. Book Compilation © 2016 Foundation for the
Sociology of Health & Illness/Blackwell Publishing Ltd.